PALLE KROEIS

Guided Meditation for Beginners

The Ultimate Journey to Inner Peace: Mastering Meditation and Mindfulness for a Balanced Life

Contents

Introduction

What is Meditation?

Meditation is an ancient practice that involves focusing the mind to achieve a state of relaxation, clarity, and heightened awareness. Originating from various cultural and religious traditions, meditation has been used for thousands of years as a tool for spiritual growth, mental clarity, and emotional well-being.

Definition and Origins

Meditation, in its simplest form, can be defined as a practice where an individual uses a technique – such as mindfulness, focusing the mind on a particular object, thought, or activity – to train attention and awareness, and achieve a mentally clear and emotionally calm and stable state. While the exact origins of meditation are hard to pinpoint, historical records indicate that it has been practiced for millennia in various parts of the world.

The earliest records of meditation come from the Hindu traditions of Vedantism around 1500 BCE. These ancient texts describe the practice of Dhyana (meditation) as a pathway to self-realization and spiritual enlightenment. Over time, meditation spread to other Eastern religions, including Buddhism and Taoism, each developing its own unique approaches and techniques.

Buddhism, which originated in India around the 5th century BCE, emphasizes meditation as a core component of its practice. The Buddha himself attained enlightenment through meditation, and he taught various forms of meditation to his disciples. Buddhist meditation practices include mindfulness (Sati) and concentration (Samadhi) techniques, which are integral to the path toward enlightenment.

In China, Taoist meditation practices emerged around the same time, focusing on inner peace and harmony with the natural world. Taoist meditation often involves breathing exercises, visualization, and movement-based practices like Tai Chi and Qigong.

Meditation also found its way into Western traditions, particularly through the influence of Greek philosophy. The writings of the Stoic philosophers, such as Marcus Aurelius and Epictetus, discuss practices similar to meditation, emphasizing self-reflection and the cultivation of inner tranquility.

Different Types of Meditation

Meditation has evolved into various forms, each with its own distinct methods and goals. Here are some of the most common types:

1. Mindfulness Meditation
   - Originating from Buddhist traditions, mindfulness meditation involves paying attention to thoughts, sensations, and feelings without

judgment. The goal is to become more aware of the present moment and develop a non-reactive awareness.

2. Transcendental Meditation
- This form of meditation involves the use of a specific mantra, repeated silently, to help the practitioner settle into a state of profound rest and relaxation, transcending ordinary thought processes.

3. Loving-Kindness Meditation (Metta)
- Practiced mainly in Buddhist traditions, loving-kindness meditation focuses on developing feelings of compassion and love for oneself and others. The practitioner silently repeats phrases such as "May I be happy, may I be well," gradually extending these wishes to others.

4. Body Scan Meditation
- Often used in mindfulness-based stress reduction (MBSR), body scan meditation involves systematically focusing attention on different parts of the body, promoting awareness and relaxation.

5. Zen Meditation (Zazen)
- A form of seated meditation from the Zen Buddhist tradition, Zazen involves focusing on the breath and observing thoughts and sensations as they arise and pass away, cultivating a deep sense of presence and clarity.

6. Guided Meditation
- In guided meditation, a teacher or guide provides instructions and visualizations, helping the practitioner achieve a meditative state. This form is especially helpful for beginners as it provides structure and support.

7. Vipassana Meditation

- Also known as "insight meditation," Vipassana aims to develop insight into the true nature of reality through focused attention and awareness of bodily sensations, thoughts, and emotions.

8. Chakra Meditation

- Rooted in the traditions of Hinduism and yoga, chakra meditation focuses on the body's energy centers (chakras) to balance and align the flow of energy.

9. Yoga Nidra

- Known as "yogic sleep," this practice involves guided meditation that leads the practitioner into a state of deep relaxation and conscious awareness between wakefulness and sleep.

Meditation practices can be broadly categorized into two main approaches: focused attention (concentration) and open monitoring (mindfulness). Focused attention meditation involves concentrating on a single object, such as the breath or a mantra, to cultivate a deep state of focus. Open monitoring meditation, on the other hand, involves observing thoughts, sensations, and emotions as they arise, promoting a state of non-judgmental awareness.

In summary, meditation is a diverse and ancient practice with a rich history across various cultures and traditions. It offers numerous benefits, ranging from physical health improvements to enhanced mental clarity and spiritual growth. Whether through mindfulness, transcendental techniques, or guided sessions, meditation provides a valuable tool for anyone seeking to cultivate a state of inner peace and well-being.

Benefits of Meditation

Meditation offers a multitude of benefits that span physical, mental, and spiritual dimensions. As a practice that encourages mindfulness and relaxation, it has been shown to improve overall well-being in various ways. Below, we delve into the primary benefits of meditation and how it can positively impact different aspects of life.

Physical Health Benefits

1. Stress Reduction

- One of the most well-documented benefits of meditation is its ability to reduce stress. By promoting relaxation and helping individuals manage their reactions to stressors, meditation can significantly lower levels of the stress hormone cortisol. This reduction in stress can lead to numerous health benefits, including improved immune function and decreased inflammation.

2. Lower Blood Pressure

- Regular meditation practice has been shown to help lower blood pressure. The relaxation response induced by meditation can reduce the strain on the heart and improve overall cardiovascular health. This benefit is particularly valuable for individuals with hypertension or those at risk of heart disease.

3. Improved Sleep

- Meditation can enhance the quality of sleep by calming the mind and reducing the anxiety that often interferes with restful sleep. Techniques such as mindfulness meditation and guided imagery can help individuals fall asleep more easily and enjoy deeper, more restorative sleep.

4. Pain Management

- Meditation has been found to be effective in managing chronic pain. By altering the perception of pain and enhancing the body's natural pain-relief mechanisms, meditation can help reduce the intensity of pain and improve the quality of life for individuals with chronic pain conditions.

5. Boosted Immune System

- Regular meditation practice can enhance the functioning of the immune system. By reducing stress and promoting relaxation, meditation helps the body maintain a state of balance and resilience, making it better equipped to fight off illnesses and infections.

Mental Health Benefits

1. Reduced Anxiety and Depression

- Meditation is a powerful tool for managing anxiety and depression. Mindfulness meditation, in particular, helps individuals become more aware of their thoughts and feelings without getting caught up in them. This awareness can reduce the impact of negative thought patterns and improve overall emotional well-being.

2. Enhanced Focus and Concentration

- Meditation improves attention span and the ability to concentrate. Techniques that involve focused attention, such as mindfulness and transcendental meditation, train the mind to stay present and focused, leading to better performance in tasks that require sustained attention.

3. Increased Emotional Resilience

- By promoting a non-judgmental awareness of thoughts and emotions, meditation helps individuals develop greater emotional resilience. This resilience allows them to navigate life's challenges with more ease and less emotional turmoil.

4. Greater Self-Awareness

- Meditation fosters a deeper understanding of oneself by encouraging introspection and self-reflection. This increased self-awareness can lead to personal growth, better decision-making, and a greater sense of purpose and fulfillment.

5. Improved Cognitive Function

- Regular meditation practice has been associated with improvements in various aspects of cognitive function, including memory, problem-solving skills, and creativity. These cognitive benefits are thought to result from the brain's increased ability to reorganize itself in response to meditation.

Spiritual Benefits

1. Inner Peace and Calm

- One of the core goals of meditation is to cultivate a sense of inner peace and calm. This state of tranquility can provide a profound sense of relief from the constant noise and chaos of daily life, allowing individuals to experience a deeper sense of contentment and well-being.

2. Connection to a Higher Purpose

- For many, meditation is a spiritual practice that enhances their connection to a higher purpose or greater reality. This sense of connection can provide meaning and direction in life, fostering a deeper sense of fulfillment and spiritual growth.

3. Enhanced Intuition

- Meditation can help individuals develop their intuition by quieting the mind and allowing deeper insights to emerge. This enhanced intuition can guide personal and professional decisions, leading to more aligned and authentic living.

4. Personal Transformation

- Through regular meditation practice, individuals often experience profound personal transformation. This transformation can manifest as increased compassion, greater empathy, and a more loving and kind disposition towards oneself and others.

5. Sense of Oneness

- Meditation can foster a sense of oneness with the universe and a feeling of interconnectedness with all living beings. This spiritual experience can lead to a greater appreciation of life and a more compassionate and altruistic approach to others.

In summary, meditation offers a comprehensive range of benefits that enhance physical health, improve mental well-being, and promote spiritual growth. Whether used as a tool for stress reduction, a method for improving focus and concentration, or a path to deeper spiritual understanding, meditation provides a valuable practice for enhancing overall quality of life. By integrating meditation into daily routines, individuals can experience these benefits and cultivate a more balanced, peaceful, and fulfilling existence.

Why Guided Meditation?

Embarking on a meditation journey can be daunting, especially for beginners. Guided meditation offers a structured and supportive entry into the practice, making it accessible and enjoyable. This section explores the reasons why guided meditation is particularly beneficial for those new to meditation, highlighting the ease of starting, the support it provides, and the ways it helps overcome common challenges.

Ease of Starting

1. Structured Approach

   - Guided meditation provides a clear and structured approach, which is particularly helpful for beginners. Instead of figuring out what to do on their own, newcomers can follow along with instructions that guide them through the process step-by-step. This structure helps demystify meditation and makes it less intimidating.

2. No Prior Knowledge Required

   - One of the biggest advantages of guided meditation is that it requires no prior knowledge or experience. Beginners can jump right in and start meditating without needing to study techniques or philosophies beforehand. The guide provides all the necessary instructions, allowing participants to focus solely on the experience.

3. Variety of Formats

   - Guided meditations come in various formats, including audio recordings, videos, and apps. This variety allows individuals to choose the format that best suits their preferences and lifestyle. Whether someone prefers listening to a soothing voice through headphones, watching a calming video, or using an interactive app, there are numerous options available.

Structure and Support

1. Professional Guidance

- Guided meditation is often led by experienced instructors or practitioners who offer their expertise and insights. This professional guidance ensures that participants are practicing correctly and effectively, maximizing the benefits of meditation. Instructors often share tips and advice that can enhance the meditation experience.

2. Consistency and Routine

- Having a guide helps establish a regular meditation routine. Scheduled sessions or daily prompts from apps can remind individuals to meditate, promoting consistency. This regularity is crucial for reaping the long-term benefits of meditation, as consistent practice helps deepen the experience and reinforces positive habits.

3. Focus and Concentration

- Beginners often struggle with maintaining focus and concentration during meditation. Guided sessions help keep the mind engaged by providing continuous direction and prompts. This can prevent the mind from wandering too much and make it easier to stay present and attentive throughout the session.

Overcoming Common Challenges

1. Handling Distractions
   - Distractions are a common challenge for new meditators. Guided meditation helps manage these distractions by offering a focal point in the form of the guide's voice. This external focus can be particularly helpful in environments where external noises or internal thoughts might otherwise disrupt the meditation.

2. Managing Restlessness
   - Many beginners experience restlessness or impatience during meditation. Guided meditation addresses this by gently leading participants through the session, offering reassurance and techniques to manage these feelings. The guide's calming presence can help individuals stay committed to the practice, even when they feel fidgety or uncomfortable.

3. Emotional Support
   - Meditation can sometimes bring up unexpected emotions. Guided meditation provides emotional support by offering a safe and controlled environment. The guide's instructions can help participants process and navigate these emotions, ensuring that they feel supported and understood throughout their meditation journey.

Enhancing the Meditation Experience

1. Themed Sessions
   - Guided meditations often focus on specific themes or goals, such as stress relief, sleep improvement, or boosting creativity. These themed sessions allow individuals to choose meditations that align with their

current needs and interests, making the practice more relevant and engaging.

2. Progressive Learning

- Many guided meditation programs are designed to progress over time, gradually introducing more advanced techniques and concepts. This progressive learning approach helps beginners build their skills and deepen their practice in a manageable and supportive way. It ensures that they continue to grow and develop their meditation practice.

3. Variety and Exploration

- Guided meditation allows individuals to explore a variety of meditation styles and techniques. This exploration can be particularly beneficial for beginners, as it helps them discover what resonates most with them. Trying different approaches can keep the practice fresh and interesting, preventing boredom and encouraging long-term commitment.

In summary, guided meditation offers an accessible, structured, and supportive way for beginners to start meditating. By providing professional guidance, helping manage common challenges, and enhancing the overall experience, guided meditation makes it easier for individuals to incorporate meditation into their lives and enjoy its numerous benefits. Whether through apps, recordings, or live sessions, guided meditation is an invaluable tool for anyone looking to embark on their meditation journey.

1

Getting Started with Guided Meditation

Understanding Guided Meditation

Guided meditation is a powerful and accessible tool for anyone interested in starting a meditation practice. Unlike other forms of meditation where one might meditate in silence or with minimal guidance, guided meditation involves a narrator or instructor who leads the practitioner through the meditation process. This section explores the fundamentals of guided meditation, explaining what it is, how it works, and why it is particularly beneficial for beginners.

Definition and Basic Concepts

Guided meditation is a type of meditation where an experienced instructor or a recorded guide provides step-by-step instructions throughout the session. The guide's role is to facilitate the meditation by offering continuous verbal support, directing the practitioner's focus, and creating a conducive environment for relaxation and mindfulness.

During a guided meditation session, the guide may focus on various elements such as breathing, bodily sensations, visualizations, or specific themes like relaxation or compassion. The guidance can be delivered in person, through audio recordings, or via meditation apps and online platforms, making it widely accessible.

Key Elements of Guided Meditation

1. The Guide's Voice
   - The guide's voice is the most distinctive feature of guided meditation. The continuous verbal instructions provide a point of focus, helping practitioners to stay engaged and anchored in the present moment. The guide's tone is typically calm and soothing, promoting a state of relaxation.

2. Structured Sessions
   - Guided meditation sessions follow a structured format, which usually includes an introduction, the main meditation practice, and a conclusion. This structure provides a clear framework, helping practitioners understand what to expect and how to proceed, making it especially useful for beginners.

3. Focused Attention
   - The guide directs the practitioner's attention to specific focal points such as the breath, a mantra, or a visualization. This focused attention helps to quiet the mind, reduce distractions, and deepen the meditation experience.

4. Thematic Meditations

- Guided meditations often revolve around specific themes or goals, such as stress relief, sleep improvement, or cultivating compassion. These thematic sessions allow practitioners to choose meditations that align with their personal needs and interests.

How Guided Meditation Works

Guided meditation works by providing a supportive framework that helps individuals focus their attention and enter a state of relaxation and mindfulness. The guide's instructions serve as an anchor, helping to keep the mind from wandering and bringing it back to the present moment whenever it strays.

Here are the typical steps involved in a guided meditation session:

1. Preparation

- The session usually begins with a brief introduction. The guide sets the tone and explains the focus of the meditation. Practitioners are encouraged to find a comfortable seated or lying position and to close their eyes if they feel comfortable doing so.

2. Relaxation

- The guide often starts with relaxation techniques, such as deep breathing or progressive muscle relaxation, to help practitioners release physical tension and prepare their minds for meditation.

3. Guided Instructions

- The main part of the session involves the guide leading the practitioner through the meditation. This can include directing attention to the breath, guiding through a body scan, suggesting visualizations, or repeating affirmations or mantras.

4. Return to Awareness

- Towards the end of the session, the guide gradually brings the practitioner back to full awareness. This may involve gently instructing them to become aware of their surroundings, wiggle their fingers and toes, and slowly open their eyes.

5. Reflection

- Some guided meditations include a brief period of reflection, where the guide encourages practitioners to take note of their experiences and any insights gained during the session.

Why Guided Meditation is Beneficial for Beginners

1. Ease of Entry

- Guided meditation offers a straightforward entry point for beginners. The continuous guidance helps reduce the uncertainty and confusion that often accompany independent meditation practice, making it easier to get started and stay committed.

2. Structured Support

- The structured nature of guided meditation provides a clear framework, which is particularly helpful for those new to meditation. Knowing that there is a set sequence to follow can reduce anxiety and increase confidence in the practice.

3. Enhanced Focus

- Beginners often struggle with maintaining focus during meditation.

Guided meditation addresses this by providing continuous verbal cues that help keep the mind anchored and reduce the tendency to become distracted.

4. Accessible Anytime, Anywhere

- With the availability of guided meditation apps and online resources, beginners can access guided sessions anytime and anywhere. This flexibility makes it easier to incorporate meditation into daily routines and find a practice that fits individual schedules.

5. Customization and Variety

- Guided meditation offers a wide range of options tailored to different needs and preferences. Whether someone is looking to reduce stress, improve sleep, or enhance creativity, there are guided meditations designed to meet those specific goals.

6. Emotional and Mental Support

- The guide's presence provides emotional and mental support, making it easier to navigate the ups and downs of meditation practice. The reassurance and encouragement from a guide can help beginners stay motivated and overcome challenges.

Conclusion

Guided meditation is an excellent starting point for anyone new to meditation. By providing structured, supportive, and accessible guidance, it helps beginners ease into the practice and experience the numerous benefits of meditation. With a variety of formats and themes available, guided meditation offers a versatile and effective way to cultivate mindfulness, relaxation, and overall well-being. As you begin your journey with guided meditation, you will find it to be a valuable tool for enhancing your quality of life and fostering a deeper sense of inner peace and balance.

Choosing the Right Environment

Creating an optimal environment for guided meditation is crucial for maximizing the benefits of your practice. A well-chosen space can enhance your ability to focus, relax, and fully immerse yourself in the meditation experience. This section provides guidance on how to select and set up an ideal environment for your meditation sessions.

Finding a Quiet Space

1. Minimize Noise

- Choose a location that is as quiet as possible. Background noise can be distracting and disrupt your focus. If you live in a noisy area, consider using noise-canceling headphones or playing soft, ambient sounds to mask external noises.

2. Dedicated Space

- If possible, designate a specific area in your home exclusively for meditation. This can help create a mental association between the space and a state of relaxation and mindfulness. It doesn't have to be a large area – a small corner or a specific room can work well.

3. Privacy

- Ensure that your meditation space offers a degree of privacy. Let household members know when you plan to meditate, so they can avoid interrupting you. A private space helps you feel more secure and allows you to fully engage in the practice without distractions.

Setting Up a Comfortable Spot

1. Comfortable Seating

- Choose a comfortable seat that allows you to maintain a relaxed but upright posture. This could be a meditation cushion (zafu), a chair, or a yoga mat. The key is to find a position that you can sustain comfortably for the duration of your meditation session.

2. Supportive Environment

- Use props like cushions, blankets, or bolsters to support your body. If sitting on the floor, a cushion under your hips can help align your spine and reduce discomfort. If using a chair, ensure your feet are flat on the ground and your back is supported.

3. Temperature and Lighting

- Adjust the temperature of your meditation space to a comfortable level. Use soft, natural lighting or dim lamps to create a calming atmosphere. Avoid harsh, bright lights that can be distracting. Candles or salt lamps can also add a soothing ambiance.

Minimizing Distractions

1. Turn Off Electronics

- Before beginning your session, turn off or silence electronic devices to prevent interruptions. This includes phones, tablets, and computers.

If using a meditation app, make sure notifications are disabled during your practice.

2. Clear Clutter

- A clutter-free environment can help promote a sense of calm and order. Remove unnecessary items from your meditation space to create a clean and serene atmosphere. This physical clarity can translate into mental clarity, aiding your meditation practice.

3. Aromatherapy

- Consider incorporating aromatherapy into your meditation environment. Essential oils like lavender, sandalwood, or chamomile can promote relaxation and enhance your meditation experience. Use a diffuser, incense, or a few drops on a tissue to introduce calming scents.

Personalizing Your Space

1. Meaningful Objects

- Decorate your meditation area with objects that have personal significance or inspire tranquility. This could include items like crystals, spiritual symbols, or artwork. These objects can serve as focal points or simply enhance the peaceful ambiance of your space.

2. Nature Elements

- Bringing elements of nature into your meditation space can create a grounding effect. Consider adding plants, flowers, or a small water feature like a fountain. Natural elements can help you feel more connected to the environment and promote a sense of inner peace.

3. Comfortable Attire

- Wear comfortable clothing that allows for easy movement and doesn't restrict your body. Loose-fitting, breathable fabrics are ideal. Being physically comfortable helps minimize distractions and allows you to focus more fully on your meditation.

Creating a Ritual

1. Consistent Practice

- Establish a routine by meditating at the same time and in the same place each day. This consistency helps build a habit and signals to your mind and body that it's time to relax and meditate.

2. Pre-Meditation Rituals

- Develop a pre-meditation ritual to prepare yourself for the practice. This could include activities like gentle stretching, deep breathing exercises, or listening to calming music. These rituals help transition your mind and body into a meditative state.

3. Post-Meditation Reflection

- After your session, take a few moments to reflect on your experience. Journaling about your meditation can help consolidate insights and track your progress. This reflection time reinforces the benefits of the practice and encourages mindful awareness throughout your day.

Conclusion

Choosing the right environment for guided meditation is a foundational step in establishing a successful practice. By selecting a quiet, comfortable, and personalized space, you create an atmosphere that supports relaxation, focus, and mindfulness. Minimizing distractions and incorporating elements that promote calmness further enhance your ability to engage deeply with your meditation. As you develop a consistent routine and incorporate pre- and post-meditation rituals, you will find that your meditation practice becomes a cherished and integral part of your daily life.

Choosing the Right Environment

Creating an optimal environment for guided meditation is crucial for maximizing the benefits of your practice. A well-chosen space can enhance your ability to focus, relax, and fully immerse yourself in the meditation experience. This section provides guidance on how to select and set up an ideal environment for your meditation sessions.

Finding a Quiet Space

1. Minimize Noise

- Choose a location that is as quiet as possible. Background noise can be distracting and disrupt your focus. If you live in a noisy area, consider using noise-canceling headphones or playing soft, ambient sounds to mask external noises.

2. Dedicated Space

- If possible, designate a specific area in your home exclusively for meditation. This can help create a mental association between the space and a state of relaxation and mindfulness. It doesn't have to be a large area – a small corner or a specific room can work well.

3. Privacy

- Ensure that your meditation space offers a degree of privacy. Let household members know when you plan to meditate, so they can avoid interrupting you. A private space helps you feel more secure and allows you to fully engage in the practice without distractions.

Setting Up a Comfortable Spot

1. Comfortable Seating

- Choose a comfortable seat that allows you to maintain a relaxed but upright posture. This could be a meditation cushion (zafu), a chair, or a yoga mat. The key is to find a position that you can sustain comfortably for the duration of your meditation session.

2. Supportive Environment

- Use props like cushions, blankets, or bolsters to support your body. If sitting on the floor, a cushion under your hips can help align your spine and reduce discomfort. If using a chair, ensure your feet are flat on the ground and your back is supported.

3. Temperature and Lighting

- Adjust the temperature of your meditation space to a comfortable level. Use soft, natural lighting or dim lamps to create a calming atmosphere. Avoid harsh, bright lights that can be distracting. Candles or salt lamps can also add a soothing ambiance.

Minimizing Distractions

1. Turn Off Electronics

- Before beginning your session, turn off or silence electronic devices to prevent interruptions. This includes phones, tablets, and computers. If using a meditation app, make sure notifications are disabled during your practice.

2. Clear Clutter

- A clutter-free environment can help promote a sense of calm and order. Remove unnecessary items from your meditation space to create a clean and serene atmosphere. This physical clarity can translate into mental clarity, aiding your meditation practice.

3. Aromatherapy

- Consider incorporating aromatherapy into your meditation environment. Essential oils like lavender, sandalwood, or chamomile can promote relaxation and enhance your meditation experience. Use a diffuser, incense, or a few drops on a tissue to introduce calming scents.

Personalizing Your Space

1. Meaningful Objects

- Decorate your meditation area with objects that have personal significance or inspire tranquility. This could include items like crystals, spiritual symbols, or artwork. These objects can serve as focal points or simply enhance the peaceful ambiance of your space.

2. Nature Elements

- Bringing elements of nature into your meditation space can create a grounding effect. Consider adding plants, flowers, or a small water feature like a fountain. Natural elements can help you feel more connected to the environment and promote a sense of inner peace.

3. Comfortable Attire

- Wear comfortable clothing that allows for easy movement and doesn't restrict your body. Loose-fitting, breathable fabrics are ideal. Being physically comfortable helps minimize distractions and allows you to focus more fully on your meditation.

Creating a Ritual

1. Consistent Practice

- Establish a routine by meditating at the same time and in the same place each day. This consistency helps build a habit and signals to your mind and body that it's time to relax and meditate.

2. Pre-Meditation Rituals

- Develop a pre-meditation ritual to prepare yourself for the practice. This could include activities like gentle stretching, deep breathing exercises, or listening to calming music. These rituals help transition your mind and body into a meditative state.

3. Post-Meditation Reflection

- After your session, take a few moments to reflect on your experience. Journaling about your meditation can help consolidate insights and track your progress. This reflection time reinforces the benefits of the practice and encourages mindful awareness throughout your day.

Conclusion

Choosing the right environment for guided meditation is a foundational step in establishing a successful practice. By selecting a quiet, comfortable, and personalized space, you create an atmosphere that supports relaxation, focus, and mindfulness. Minimizing distractions and incorporating elements that promote calmness further enhance your ability to engage deeply with your meditation. As you develop a consistent routine and incorporate pre- and post-meditation rituals, you will find that your meditation practice becomes a cherished and integral part of your daily life.

Tools and Resources

To embark on a successful guided meditation journey, having the right tools and resources can make a significant difference. These can enhance your practice, provide guidance, and help you stay committed. This section outlines essential tools and resources that can support your guided meditation practice.

Meditation Apps and Websites

1. Popular Meditation Apps
  - Headspace: Known for its user-friendly interface and extensive library of guided meditations, Headspace offers sessions tailored to various needs, including stress reduction, sleep improvement, and focus enhancement.
  - Calm: Calm provides a wide range of guided meditations, sleep

stories, and calming music. It also offers programs for beginners and more advanced practitioners.

- Insight Timer: This app boasts a vast collection of free guided meditations from various teachers around the world. It also features a customizable meditation timer and community features to connect with other meditators.

2. Meditation Websites

- Mindful.org: This website offers a wealth of resources, including guided meditations, articles, and tips for integrating mindfulness into daily life.

- Tara Brach: Tara Brach's website provides free access to numerous guided meditations and talks focused on mindfulness and compassion.

- UCLA Mindful Awareness Research Center: This site offers free guided meditations and mindfulness resources developed by the University of California, Los Angeles.

Music and Nature Sounds

1. Meditation Music

- Listening to soothing music can enhance your meditation experience by creating a relaxing atmosphere. Look for instrumental music, ambient sounds, or binaural beats designed for meditation. Apps like Calm and Insight Timer offer extensive libraries of meditation music.

2. Nature Sounds

- Nature sounds such as flowing water, bird songs, or gentle rain can help create a calming environment and aid in relaxation. Many meditation apps include nature soundscapes, or you can find free recordings on platforms like YouTube and Spotify.

Essential Equipment

1. Meditation Cushion (Zafu)

- A meditation cushion helps maintain a comfortable and stable seated posture, which is crucial for longer meditation sessions. It supports the hips and aligns the spine, reducing discomfort and promoting relaxation.

2. Meditation Mat (Zabuton)

- Placing a meditation mat under your cushion can provide additional comfort by cushioning your knees and ankles. This is especially useful if you meditate on a hard surface.

3. Chair or Bench

- If sitting on the floor is uncomfortable, consider using a chair or a meditation bench. Ensure that your feet are flat on the ground and your back is supported. The goal is to maintain an upright posture without straining.

Books and Reading Material

1. Introduction to Meditation Books

- "The Miracle of Mindfulness" by Thich Nhat Hanh: This classic book provides practical advice and exercises for developing mindfulness in everyday life.
- "Wherever You Go, There You Are" by Jon Kabat-Zinn: A comprehensive guide to mindfulness meditation, offering insights and techniques for incorporating meditation into daily routines.

2. Deepening Your Practice

- "Radical Acceptance" by Tara Brach: This book explores how mindfulness and self-compassion can help you embrace your true self and overcome emotional challenges.

- "The Untethered Soul" by Michael A. Singer: A deeper exploration of consciousness and meditation, offering insights into how to achieve inner freedom and peace.

Online Courses and Workshops

1. Beginner Courses

- Many meditation apps and websites offer structured courses for beginners. For example, Headspace and Calm provide introductory programs that guide you through the basics of meditation.

2. Advanced Training

- For those looking to deepen their practice, consider enrolling in online courses or attending workshops led by experienced meditation teachers. Websites like Mindful.org and the Insight Meditation Society offer a variety of courses and retreats.

3. Live Sessions and Webinars

- Participating in live meditation sessions or webinars can provide real-time guidance and an opportunity to connect with instructors and fellow meditators. Look for events hosted by reputable meditation centers or instructors.

Journaling Tools

1. Meditation Journal

- Keeping a meditation journal can help you track your progress, reflect on your experiences, and set intentions for your practice. Note any insights, challenges, or changes you observe over time.

2. Guided Journals

- Consider using a guided journal designed specifically for meditation practitioners. These journals often include prompts, tips, and spaces for reflection, making it easier to maintain a consistent journaling practice.

Community and Support

1. Meditation Groups

- Joining a local or online meditation group can provide support, accountability, and a sense of community. Many apps and websites have built-in community features where you can connect with other meditators.

2. Social Media and Forums

- Engage with meditation communities on social media platforms like Facebook, Reddit, or Instagram. These communities offer a space to share experiences, ask questions, and receive encouragement.

Conclusion

Equipping yourself with the right tools and resources can significantly enhance your guided meditation practice. Whether through meditation apps, music, essential equipment, or community support, these resources provide the guidance and structure needed to develop a consistent and effective meditation routine. By exploring and utilizing these tools, you can create a supportive environment that fosters relaxation, mindfulness, and personal growth.

2

Preparing for Your First Session

Setting Your Intention

Setting an intention is a powerful way to begin your meditation practice. It provides direction, purpose, and focus, helping you stay motivated and centered throughout your meditation journey. This section explores the importance of setting an intention, how to do it effectively, and the benefits it can bring to your guided meditation practice.

Importance of Setting an Intention

1. Provides Focus and Clarity

- Setting an intention helps you focus your mind and provides clarity about what you hope to achieve with your meditation practice. It gives your session a sense of purpose, making it easier to stay engaged and present.

2. Enhances Motivation

- Having a clear intention can boost your motivation to meditate regularly. When you understand why you are meditating and what you hope to gain, it becomes easier to commit to your practice and make it a consistent part of your routine.

3. Guides Your Practice

- An intention serves as a guiding principle for your meditation. Whether it's cultivating mindfulness, reducing stress, or fostering compassion, your intention can shape the focus and direction of your sessions.

4. Promotes Mindfulness

- Setting an intention encourages mindfulness by prompting you to reflect on your goals and desires. This reflection can deepen your self-awareness and help you stay connected to your inner experiences during meditation.

How to Set an Intention

1. Reflect on Your Goals

- Take some time to reflect on why you want to meditate. What are you hoping to achieve? What aspects of your life do you want to improve? Your goals might include reducing anxiety, improving focus, enhancing emotional well-being, or simply finding more peace in your daily life.

2. Be Specific and Realistic

- When setting your intention, be specific and realistic about what you want to achieve. Instead of a vague intention like "I want to be happier," consider something more specific like "I intend to practice gratitude and notice the positive aspects of my life."

3. Keep It Positive

- Frame your intention in a positive light. Focus on what you want to bring into your life rather than what you want to eliminate. For example, instead of saying "I want to stop feeling anxious," set an intention like "I intend to cultivate calm and relaxation."

4. Write It Down

- Writing down your intention can reinforce your commitment and make it feel more tangible. Keep your written intention somewhere visible, such as in a journal, on a sticky note, or as a reminder on your phone.

5. Repeat Your Intention

- At the beginning of each meditation session, take a moment to silently repeat your intention. This practice helps to center your mind and remind you of your purpose for meditating.

Examples of Intentions

1. Mindfulness

- "I intend to be fully present and aware in each moment."
- "I intend to observe my thoughts and feelings without judgment."

2. Stress Reduction

- "I intend to release tension and cultivate inner peace."
- "I intend to let go of stress and embrace relaxation."

3. Emotional Well-Being

- "I intend to nurture self-compassion and kindness."
- "I intend to open my heart to love and forgiveness."

4. Focus and Clarity

- "I intend to enhance my concentration and mental clarity."
- "I intend to stay focused and grounded in the present moment."

5. Gratitude and Positivity

- "I intend to practice gratitude and appreciate the blessings in my life."
- "I intend to cultivate a positive outlook and embrace joy."

Benefits of Setting an Intention

1. Enhanced Meditation Experience

- Having a clear intention can make your meditation sessions more meaningful and rewarding. It provides a sense of direction and purpose, helping you stay engaged and motivated.

2. Personal Growth

- Setting intentions encourages self-reflection and personal growth. As you work towards your goals, you may gain insights into your thoughts, behaviors, and patterns, leading to greater self-awareness and transformation.

3. Improved Focus and Discipline

- An intention acts as an anchor, helping you maintain focus and discipline in your practice. It can remind you why you started meditating and keep you committed to your journey, even on days when it feels challenging.

4. Greater Mindfulness and Presence

- By setting an intention, you cultivate a more mindful and present approach to life. This mindfulness can extend beyond your meditation sessions, helping you stay connected to the present moment and navigate daily challenges with greater ease.

5. Emotional and Mental Well-Being

- Intentions that focus on emotional and mental well-being can lead to profound positive changes. Whether it's fostering self-compassion, reducing stress, or enhancing positivity, a clear intention can help you create a more balanced and fulfilling life.

Conclusion

Setting an intention is a vital step in preparing for your guided meditation practice. It provides focus, motivation, and a sense of purpose, enhancing the overall meditation experience. By reflecting on your goals, being specific and positive, and integrating your intention into your practice, you can cultivate mindfulness, personal growth, and emotional well-being. As you continue your meditation journey, let your intention guide and inspire you, helping you achieve a deeper sense of peace and fulfillment.

Basic Breathing Techniques

Breathing is a fundamental aspect of meditation. It serves as a powerful tool to anchor your mind, enhance relaxation, and bring your focus to the present moment. Learning and practicing basic breathing techniques can significantly improve your guided meditation experience. This section introduces several foundational breathing techniques that are simple yet effective for beginners.

The Importance of Breath in Meditation

1. Anchoring the Mind

- Focusing on the breath helps to anchor the mind, reducing the tendency to become distracted by thoughts. It provides a constant, rhythmic point of attention that can bring you back to the present moment whenever your mind wanders.

2. Promoting Relaxation

- Controlled breathing activates the body's relaxation response, lowering stress levels, reducing tension, and promoting a state of calm. This physiological effect is crucial for achieving a meditative state.

3. Enhancing Mindfulness

- Mindfulness is the practice of being fully present and aware. By observing the breath, you cultivate a heightened sense of mindfulness, which can extend beyond meditation into daily life.

Basic Breathing Techniques

1. Diaphragmatic Breathing (Belly Breathing)
- Diaphragmatic breathing, or belly breathing, involves deep breaths that fully engage the diaphragm. This technique maximizes oxygen intake and promotes relaxation.

How to Practice Diaphragmatic Breathing:
- Sit or lie down in a comfortable position.
- Place one hand on your chest and the other on your belly.
- Take a slow, deep breath in through your nose, allowing your belly to rise as you fill your lungs with air.
- Exhale slowly through your mouth, feeling your belly fall as you release the air.
- Focus on the rise and fall of your belly, and try to keep your chest relatively still.
- Repeat for several breaths, maintaining a slow and steady rhythm.

2. Box Breathing (Four-Square Breathing)
- Box breathing is a simple and effective technique that involves breathing in a square pattern. It helps to regulate your breathing and calm the mind.

How to Practice Box Breathing:
- Sit comfortably with your back straight.
- Inhale through your nose for a count of four.
- Hold your breath for a count of four.
- Exhale slowly through your mouth for a count of four.
- Hold your breath again for a count of four.
- Repeat the cycle for several minutes, maintaining a steady and even rhythm.

3. Alternate Nostril Breathing (Nadi Shodhana)

- Alternate nostril breathing is a yogic breathing technique that balances the flow of energy in the body and promotes a sense of calm and clarity.

How to Practice Alternate Nostril Breathing:

- Sit comfortably with your spine straight and shoulders relaxed.
- Place your left hand on your left knee, and bring your right hand up to your nose.
- Use your right thumb to close your right nostril.
- Inhale slowly and deeply through your left nostril.
- Close your left nostril with your right ring finger, and open your right nostril.
- Exhale slowly and completely through your right nostril.
- Inhale through your right nostril, then close it with your right thumb.
- Open your left nostril and exhale through the left nostril.
- This completes one cycle. Repeat for several cycles, maintaining a smooth and steady breath.

4. 4-7-8 Breathing

- The 4-7-8 breathing technique is a powerful method for calming the nervous system and reducing stress. It involves specific timing for inhaling, holding the breath, and exhaling.

How to Practice 4-7-8 Breathing:

- Sit or lie down in a comfortable position with your back straight.
- Place the tip of your tongue against the ridge of tissue just behind your upper front teeth and keep it there throughout the exercise.
- Exhale completely through your mouth, making a whooshing sound.

- Close your mouth and inhale quietly through your nose for a count of four.
- Hold your breath for a count of seven.
- Exhale completely through your mouth, making a whooshing sound, for a count of eight.
- This completes one breath. Repeat the cycle for four breaths initially, and gradually increase as you become more comfortable.

5. Mindful Breathing

- Mindful breathing involves paying close attention to the natural rhythm and sensation of your breath without trying to change it. It is a fundamental practice in mindfulness meditation.

How to Practice Mindful Breathing:

- Sit comfortably with your back straight and hands resting on your lap.
- Close your eyes and bring your attention to your breath.
- Notice the sensation of the air entering and leaving your nostrils.
- Feel the rise and fall of your chest or abdomen with each breath.
- If your mind wanders, gently bring your focus back to the sensation of your breath.
- Continue for several minutes, maintaining a gentle and non-judgmental awareness of your breath.

Integrating Breathing Techniques into Guided Meditation

1. Starting with Breath Awareness

- Begin your guided meditation session with a few minutes of focused breathing. This helps to settle your mind and body, preparing you for deeper meditation.

2. Using Breath as an Anchor

- Throughout the guided meditation, use your breath as an anchor. Whenever your mind starts to wander, gently return your focus to your breath.

3. Ending with Deep Breaths

- Conclude your meditation session with a few deep, calming breaths. This helps to transition from the meditative state back to your daily activities with a sense of calm and clarity.

Conclusion

Mastering basic breathing techniques is an essential step in preparing for your guided meditation sessions. These techniques provide a foundation for relaxation, focus, and mindfulness, enhancing the overall meditation experience. By incorporating diaphragmatic breathing, box breathing, alternate nostril breathing, 4-7-8 breathing, and mindful breathing into your practice, you can cultivate a deeper sense of peace and presence. As you become more comfortable with these techniques, you will find that your ability to enter and maintain a meditative state improves, bringing greater benefits to your guided meditation journey.

Mindfulness and Awareness

Mindfulness and awareness are core components of a successful meditation practice. They involve paying attention to the present moment with a non-judgmental attitude and cultivating a heightened sense of awareness of your thoughts, feelings, and surroundings. This section explores the concepts of mindfulness and awareness, their importance in guided meditation, and practical techniques to develop these skills.

Understanding Mindfulness

1. Definition of Mindfulness

- Mindfulness is the practice of deliberately focusing your attention on the present moment and accepting it without judgment. It involves being fully aware of your thoughts, emotions, bodily sensations, and environment, allowing you to experience each moment as it unfolds.

2. Benefits of Mindfulness

- Reduces Stress: Mindfulness helps to reduce stress by encouraging a calm and relaxed state of mind. By focusing on the present, you can let go of worries about the past or future.

- Enhances Emotional Regulation: Practicing mindfulness can improve your ability to manage and regulate emotions, leading to greater emotional stability and resilience.

- Improves Concentration: Mindfulness enhances your ability to concentrate and stay focused on tasks, which can improve productivity and performance.

- Promotes Well-being: Regular mindfulness practice has been shown to increase overall well-being, leading to a greater sense of happiness and fulfillment.

Understanding Awareness

1. Definition of Awareness

- Awareness is the ability to consciously perceive and observe your internal and external experiences. It involves noticing your thoughts, emotions, and physical sensations without becoming attached to them or reacting automatically.

2. Role of Awareness in Meditation

- Awareness is a crucial aspect of meditation as it allows you to observe your mental and emotional states objectively. By developing awareness, you can recognize patterns, habits, and automatic reactions, which can lead to greater self-understanding and personal growth.

Techniques to Develop Mindfulness and Awareness

1. Mindful Breathing

- Practice: Focus on your breath as it flows in and out of your body. Notice the sensation of the air entering and leaving your nostrils, the rise and fall of your chest or abdomen, and the rhythm of your breathing.
- Benefits: Mindful breathing anchors your attention to the present moment, calming the mind and enhancing awareness.

2. Body Scan Meditation

- Practice: Lie down or sit comfortably and bring your attention to different parts of your body, starting from your toes and moving up to your head. Notice any sensations, tension, or areas of relaxation.
- Benefits: Body scan meditation increases awareness of bodily sensations and helps to release physical tension, promoting relaxation.

3. Mindful Observation

- Practice: Choose an object, such as a flower, a piece of fruit, or a candle flame, and observe it closely. Notice its colors, textures, shapes, and any other details without judgment.

- Benefits: Mindful observation enhances your ability to focus and appreciate the details of the present moment, fostering a deeper sense of awareness.

4. Mindful Listening

- Practice: Listen attentively to the sounds around you, whether it's the sound of nature, music, or a conversation. Pay attention to the quality, pitch, and rhythm of the sounds without forming judgments or reactions.

- Benefits: Mindful listening improves your ability to stay present during conversations and enhances your overall auditory awareness.

5. Thought and Emotion Observation

- Practice: Sit quietly and observe your thoughts and emotions as they arise. Notice them without getting caught up in them or trying to change them. Acknowledge their presence and let them pass naturally.

- Benefits: Observing thoughts and emotions without judgment helps you develop a non-reactive awareness, reducing emotional reactivity and promoting mental clarity.

Incorporating Mindfulness and Awareness into Guided Meditation

1. Starting with Mindfulness

- Begin your guided meditation session with a few minutes of mindful breathing or a body scan. This sets a foundation of mindfulness and helps you transition into a meditative state.

2. Maintaining Awareness

- Throughout the guided meditation, maintain a gentle awareness of your breath, bodily sensations, or the guide's instructions. If your mind wanders, gently bring your focus back to the present moment.

3. Ending with Reflection

- Conclude your session with a brief period of reflection. Notice how you feel physically, emotionally, and mentally. Reflect on any insights or experiences that arose during the meditation.

Practical Tips for Developing Mindfulness and Awareness

1. Regular Practice

- Consistency is key to developing mindfulness and awareness. Incorporate these practices into your daily routine, even if it's just for a few minutes each day.

2. Patience and Compassion

- Approach your practice with patience and self-compassion. It's normal for your mind to wander or for distractions to arise. Gently guide your focus back to the present without judgment.

3. Integrate into Daily Activities

- Practice mindfulness and awareness in everyday activities, such as eating, walking, or washing dishes. Pay attention to the sensations, thoughts, and emotions that arise during these activities.

4. Use Reminders

- Set reminders on your phone or place sticky notes in visible areas to prompt you to practice mindfulness throughout the day. These reminders can help reinforce your commitment to staying present.

Conclusion

Developing mindfulness and awareness is essential for a successful guided meditation practice. These skills allow you to stay present, reduce stress, and gain deeper insights into your thoughts and emotions. By practicing techniques such as mindful breathing, body scan meditation, mindful observation, mindful listening, and thought and emotion observation, you can cultivate a heightened sense of awareness and bring greater mindfulness into your daily life. As you prepare for your first guided meditation session, integrating mindfulness and awareness will enhance your ability to relax, focus, and fully engage with the practice.

3

The First Guided Meditation

Selecting Your First Guided Meditation

Choosing your first guided meditation is an important step in beginning your meditation journey. With numerous options available, it's essential to find a guided meditation that resonates with you and aligns with your goals. This section will help you understand how to select the right guided meditation to start with, ensuring a positive and rewarding experience.

Understanding Your Goals

1. Identify Your Purpose

- Before selecting a guided meditation, take a moment to reflect on why you want to meditate. Are you looking to reduce stress, improve sleep, enhance focus, or cultivate mindfulness? Understanding your primary motivation will help you choose a meditation that aligns with your needs.

2. Set Specific Goals

   - Once you've identified your purpose, set specific goals for your meditation practice. For example, if your aim is to reduce stress, your goal might be to feel more relaxed and centered after each session. Clear goals can guide your choice and help you measure your progress.

Types of Guided Meditations

1. Mindfulness Meditation

   - Focuses on developing present-moment awareness and observing thoughts and sensations without judgment. Ideal for beginners who want to cultivate mindfulness and reduce stress.

2. Body Scan Meditation

   - Guides you through paying attention to different parts of your body, promoting relaxation and bodily awareness. This type is excellent for releasing physical tension and fostering a mind-body connection.

3. Loving-Kindness Meditation

   - Involves generating feelings of compassion and kindness towards oneself and others. Perfect for those looking to enhance emotional well-being and develop a positive mindset.

4. Visualization Meditation

   - Uses guided imagery to create a mental picture of calming or inspiring scenes. Suitable for individuals who find visual stimuli helpful in achieving relaxation and focus.

5. Breath-Focused Meditation

   - Centers on mindful breathing techniques to anchor your attention and calm the mind. Great for beginners who want to learn to use their breath as a tool for relaxation and concentration.

6. Mantra Meditation

- Involves the repetition of a word or phrase to aid concentration and achieve a meditative state. Ideal for those who prefer a structured focus during meditation.

Choosing the Right Length

1. Short Sessions (5-10 minutes)

- Ideal for beginners who are just starting and may find it challenging to sit for longer periods. Short sessions are also great for busy schedules or as a quick mental reset during the day.

2. Medium Sessions (10-20 minutes)

- Suitable for those who have a bit more time and are ready to deepen their practice. Medium-length sessions provide a balance between accessibility and depth.

3. Long Sessions (20-60 minutes)

- Best for individuals who are comfortable with longer periods of meditation and want to explore more profound states of relaxation and mindfulness. Long sessions are often used for in-depth exploration and significant personal growth.

Finding Quality Guided Meditations

1. Trusted Sources

- Look for guided meditations from reputable sources, such as well-known meditation teachers, established meditation apps, and reputable websites. Trusted sources ensure that the guidance provided is reliable and effective.

2. User Reviews

- Check user reviews and ratings to see what others have experienced with the guided meditation. Positive feedback can indicate a valuable and well-received meditation session.

3. Sample Different Guides

- Explore different guides and instructors to find a voice and style that resonates with you. Everyone has unique preferences, and finding a guide whose voice and approach you find calming and encouraging can enhance your experience.

Recommended Platforms and Resources

1. Meditation Apps

- Headspace: Offers a variety of guided meditations for different goals, such as stress relief, sleep improvement, and mindfulness. The app also provides structured programs for beginners.
- Calm: Known for its soothing voiceovers and diverse meditation topics, Calm offers guided sessions for relaxation, focus, and emotional well-being.
- Insight Timer: Features thousands of free guided meditations from various teachers, along with a customizable meditation timer

and community features.

2. Online Platforms

- YouTube: A vast resource for free guided meditations. Channels like The Honest Guys, Michael Sealey, and Tara Brach offer high-quality sessions.

- Mindful.org: Provides a collection of guided meditations, articles, and resources for mindfulness and meditation practice.

3. Books and Audio Guides

- "The Miracle of Mindfulness" by Thich Nhat Hanh: Offers practical mindfulness exercises and guided meditations.

- "Wherever You Go, There You Are" by Jon Kabat-Zinn: Includes mindfulness meditation practices and guidance for integrating mindfulness into daily life.

Preparing for Your First Session

1. Set Up Your Environment

- Choose a quiet, comfortable space where you won't be disturbed. Ensure you have a comfortable seat or cushion, and consider using headphones to minimize distractions.

2. Gather Necessary Tools

- If you're using a meditation app or an audio guide, make sure your device is charged and you have any necessary accessories, such as headphones or a speaker.

3. Create a Routine

- Establish a regular time for your meditation practice, whether it's in the morning, during a lunch break, or before bed. Consistency helps build a habit and enhances the benefits of meditation.

Conclusion

Selecting your first guided meditation is an exciting step towards cultivating a regular meditation practice. By understanding your goals, exploring different types of meditations, choosing the right length, and utilizing trusted resources, you can find a guided meditation that suits your needs and preferences. As you prepare for your first session, remember to set up a comfortable environment and establish a routine that supports your practice. With the right guidance and preparation, you'll be well on your way to experiencing the profound benefits of guided meditation.

What to Expect

Embarking on your first guided meditation session can be an exciting and transformative experience. However, it's helpful to know what to expect so you can approach the practice with an open mind and realistic expectations. This section will walk you through the typical experiences and sensations you might encounter during your first guided meditation session.

Common Experiences

1. Initial Discomfort

- It's normal to feel some initial discomfort, both physically and mentally. You might find it challenging to sit still or maintain a comfortable posture. Your mind may also resist settling down, leading to restlessness or frustration.

2. Physical Sensations

- During meditation, you might notice various physical sensations such as tingling, warmth, or slight tension in different parts of your body. These sensations are normal and usually subside as you become more accustomed to the practice.

3. Wandering Thoughts

- A common experience for beginners is the frequent wandering of thoughts. Your mind may drift to past events, future plans, or random thoughts. This is a normal part of meditation. The key is to gently bring your focus back to the guide's instructions or your chosen point of focus.

4. Emotional Responses

- Meditation can sometimes bring up unexpected emotions. You might feel a sense of calm, joy, or even sadness and frustration. Acknowledging these emotions without judgment is an important part of the practice.

5. Moments of Stillness

- Amidst the distractions and wandering thoughts, you may experience brief moments of stillness and clarity. These moments can feel deeply peaceful and affirm the benefits of the practice.

Physical Sensations

1. Relaxation and Tension Release

- As you follow the guided meditation, you might feel a gradual release of physical tension. This can lead to a sense of relaxation and ease in your body. Focus on these sensations to deepen your relaxation.

2. Breath Awareness

- Paying attention to your breath can heighten your awareness of its rhythm and depth. You might notice how your breath affects different parts of your body, such as the rise and fall of your chest or the expansion of your abdomen.

3. Posture Adjustments

- During meditation, you may need to make small adjustments to your posture to stay comfortable. Ensure that these movements are gentle and mindful to maintain your meditative state.

Emotional Responses

1. Calm and Contentment

- Many beginners report feelings of calm and contentment during and after meditation. This emotional state arises from the relaxation and mindfulness cultivated during the practice.

2. Emotional Release

- Meditation can sometimes trigger an emotional release, bringing unresolved feelings to the surface. This can be therapeutic, allowing you to process and let go of these emotions.

3. Increased Awareness

- You may become more aware of your habitual thought patterns and emotional responses. This increased awareness can lead to greater self-understanding and emotional regulation.

Mental Challenges

1. Restlessness

- It's common to feel restless or impatient, especially if you're not used to sitting still for extended periods. Recognize this restlessness as a normal part of the process and try to gently refocus on the guided instructions.

2. Doubt and Judgment

- You might experience self-doubt or judge yourself for not meditating "correctly." Remember that meditation is a practice, and it's okay to have these thoughts. Accept them without judgment and return your focus to the meditation.

3. Difficulty Focusing

- Maintaining focus can be challenging, particularly in the beginning. Your mind might wander frequently. Each time it does, gently bring your attention back to the guide's voice or your breath. Over time, your ability to focus will improve.

Positive Experiences

1. Sense of Presence

- One of the key benefits of meditation is the cultivation of a sense of presence. You might find yourself becoming more aware of the present moment, experiencing it fully without distraction.

2. Inner Peace

- Many practitioners report a deep sense of inner peace and tranquility during and after meditation. This peaceful state arises from the mindful awareness and relaxation fostered by the practice.

3. Increased Clarity

- As you meditate, you may gain insights into your thoughts and emotions, leading to increased mental clarity. This clarity can help you understand yourself better and make more mindful decisions.

After the Meditation

1. Gradual Transition

- After your guided meditation session, take a few moments to transition back to your regular activities. Open your eyes slowly, stretch gently, and take note of how you feel.

2. Reflection

- Spend a few minutes reflecting on your experience. You might want to jot down any insights or notable experiences in a meditation journal. This reflection can help reinforce the benefits of your practice and track your progress over time.

3. Carry the Mindfulness Forward

- Try to carry the mindfulness and calm you cultivated during meditation into the rest of your day. This can enhance your overall well-being and help you integrate the benefits of meditation into your daily life.

Conclusion

Understanding what to expect during your first guided meditation can help you approach the practice with an open and accepting mindset. Remember that it's normal to experience discomfort, wandering thoughts, and emotional responses. With patience and consistent practice, you'll likely find that these challenges diminish and the positive effects of meditation become more pronounced. By recognizing and embracing the range of experiences that come with guided meditation, you set the stage for a fulfilling and transformative practice.

Post-Meditation Reflection

Reflecting on your meditation experience after each session is an essential part of developing a deeper understanding of your practice and its effects on your mind and body. Post-meditation reflection helps you consolidate your experiences, gain insights, and track your progress over time. This section will guide you through the process of reflecting on your meditation session and offer practical tips to enhance your post-meditation practice.

The Importance of Reflection

1. Deepens Understanding

- Reflecting on your meditation session allows you to deepen your understanding of your experiences. It helps you recognize patterns, identify areas of growth, and become more aware of how meditation affects your mental and emotional states.

2. Enhances Learning

- By reflecting on what worked well and what challenges you faced, you can learn more about your practice and how to improve it. This continuous learning process enhances the effectiveness of your meditation over time.

3. Promotes Mindfulness

- Post-meditation reflection is a form of mindfulness in itself. It encourages you to stay present and aware of your experiences, fostering a greater sense of mindfulness throughout your day.

How to Reflect on Your Meditation Session

1. Find a Quiet Space

- After your meditation session, find a quiet and comfortable space where you can sit and reflect without distractions. This helps maintain the calm and focused state achieved during meditation.

2. Take Your Time

- Allow yourself sufficient time for reflection. Rushing through this process can undermine its benefits. Spend a few minutes in quiet contemplation before you start writing or recording your thoughts.

3. Focus on Key Areas

- When reflecting, consider focusing on the following key areas:
- Physical Sensations: Notice any physical sensations you experienced during meditation. Were there areas of tension or relaxation? How did your body feel throughout the session?
- Emotional Responses: Reflect on any emotions that arose during meditation. Did you feel calm, anxious, joyful, or frustrated? How did you respond to these emotions?
- Mental Activity: Consider the activity of your mind. Were your thoughts racing, or did you experience moments of stillness and clarity? How often did your mind wander, and how did you bring it back to focus?
- Breath Awareness: Pay attention to your breath. How did focusing on your breath impact your meditation experience? Did you notice any changes in your breathing patterns?

4. Use a Journal

- Keeping a meditation journal is a valuable tool for post-meditation reflection. Writing down your experiences can help you organize your thoughts and track your progress over time. Include details such as the date, duration of the session, and any specific insights or challenges.

5. Ask Reflective Questions

- Use reflective questions to guide your journaling. Some examples include:
- What was the most noticeable sensation or thought during the session?
- How did I feel at the beginning of the meditation compared to the end?
- What challenges did I face, and how did I address them?
- What positive effects did I notice after the meditation?

- How can I apply the insights gained from this session to my daily life?

Benefits of Post-Meditation Reflection

1. Increased Self-Awareness

- Regular reflection enhances self-awareness by helping you understand your thoughts, emotions, and behaviors better. This increased awareness can lead to more mindful decision-making and a greater sense of control over your mental and emotional states.

2. Improved Practice

- By identifying what works well and what doesn't, you can make informed adjustments to your meditation practice. This continuous improvement can lead to more effective and fulfilling meditation sessions.

3. Emotional Processing

- Reflection provides an opportunity to process any emotions that arose during meditation. Acknowledging and understanding these emotions can lead to emotional healing and greater emotional resilience.

4. Enhanced Mindfulness

- The act of reflecting on your meditation practice reinforces mindfulness. It encourages you to stay present and aware of your experiences, both during meditation and in your daily life.

Tips for Effective Post-Meditation Reflection

1. Be Honest and Non-Judgmental

- Approach your reflection with honesty and without judgment. Accept your experiences as they are, without labeling them as good or bad. This non-judgmental attitude fosters a more compassionate and open mindset.

2. Stay Consistent

- Make reflection a regular part of your meditation practice. Consistency is key to reaping the benefits of post-meditation reflection. Try to reflect after each session, even if it's just for a few minutes.

3. Share Your Experiences

- If you feel comfortable, consider sharing your meditation experiences with a trusted friend, meditation group, or teacher. Sharing can provide additional insights and support, and it can help you stay motivated and engaged with your practice.

4. Use Visual Aids

- Incorporate visual aids such as charts or graphs to track your progress over time. Seeing your growth and changes visually can be motivating and provide a clear picture of how your practice is evolving.

Conclusion

Post-meditation reflection is a vital component of a successful meditation practice. It deepens your understanding, enhances learning, and promotes mindfulness. By taking the time to reflect on your experiences, you can gain valuable insights, improve your practice, and cultivate greater self-awareness and emotional resilience. Whether through journaling, asking reflective questions, or sharing your experiences with others, post-meditation reflection can help you make the most of your guided meditation journey.

4

Deepening Your Practice

Exploring Different Styles

As you become more comfortable with guided meditation, you may find it beneficial to explore different styles to deepen your practice and discover what resonates best with you. Each meditation style offers unique techniques and benefits, allowing you to tailor your practice to your specific needs and goals. This section introduces various meditation styles, providing an overview of their approaches and advantages.

1. Mindfulness Meditation

1. Overview

- Mindfulness meditation involves paying attention to the present moment with an attitude of openness and non-judgment. It encourages awareness of thoughts, feelings, and sensations as they arise, without becoming attached to them.

2. Techniques

- Breath Awareness: Focus on the breath, noticing each inhalation and exhalation. When the mind wanders, gently bring it back to the breath.

- Body Scan: Slowly direct attention to different parts of the body, observing any sensations without judgment.

- Open Monitoring: Observe thoughts and feelings as they come and go, maintaining a non-reactive stance.

3. Benefits

- Reduces stress and anxiety
- Improves focus and concentration
- Enhances emotional regulation
- Increases self-awareness

2. Loving-Kindness Meditation (Metta)

1. Overview

- Loving-kindness meditation focuses on developing feelings of compassion, love, and goodwill towards oneself and others. It involves silently repeating phrases that express positive wishes.

2. Techniques

- Phrases: Repeat phrases such as "May I be happy, may I be healthy, may I be safe, may I live with ease." Gradually extend these wishes to others, including loved ones, neutral people, and even those with whom you have difficulties.

- Visualization: Visualize yourself and others surrounded by a warm, loving light as you repeat the phrases.

3. Benefits
- Increases compassion and empathy
- Reduces negative emotions
- Enhances social connections
- Promotes emotional healing

3. Body Scan Meditation

1. Overview
- Body scan meditation involves systematically focusing attention on different parts of the body. It promotes relaxation and helps develop a deeper connection with bodily sensations.

2. Techniques
- Progressive Attention: Starting from the toes and moving upwards, or vice versa, focus on each body part, noticing any sensations of tension, relaxation, or neutrality.
- Breath Integration: Combine the body scan with deep, mindful breathing to enhance relaxation.

3. Benefits
- Reduces physical tension and pain
- Improves body awareness
- Enhances relaxation and stress relief
- Promotes mindful presence

4. Visualization Meditation

1. Overview

- Visualization meditation uses mental imagery to create a serene and positive experience. This technique can be used to achieve relaxation, focus, and specific goals.

2. Techniques

- Guided Imagery: Follow the guide's instructions to visualize calming scenes, such as a peaceful beach, a lush forest, or a warm, sunny meadow.

- Goal Visualization: Visualize yourself achieving specific goals, such as excelling in a task, feeling confident, or overcoming a challenge.

3. Benefits

- Enhances relaxation and stress reduction
- Boosts creativity and focus
- Helps achieve personal goals
- Strengthens mental imagery skills

5. Breath-Focused Meditation

1. Overview

- Breath-focused meditation centers on the breath as the primary point of focus. It is a simple yet powerful technique for cultivating mindfulness and relaxation.

2. Techniques

- Counting Breaths: Count each breath cycle (inhalation and exhalation) up to a certain number, then start over.

- Deep Breathing: Practice deep, diaphragmatic breathing to promote relaxation.

- Alternate Nostril Breathing: Use a specific technique to alternate breathing through each nostril, balancing the breath.

3. Benefits
- Enhances focus and concentration
- Reduces stress and anxiety
- Improves respiratory health
- **Promotes relaxation and mindfulness**

6. Mantra Meditation

1. Overview
- Mantra meditation involves the repetition of a word, phrase, or sound to aid concentration and achieve a meditative state. Mantras can be spoken aloud or silently.

2. Techniques
- Choosing a Mantra: Select a meaningful word or phrase, such as "Om," "Peace," or "I am calm."
- Repetition: Repeat the mantra rhythmically, focusing on the sound and vibration. If your mind wanders, gently bring it back to the mantra.

3. Benefits
- Improves concentration and focus
- Enhances mental clarity
- Promotes a sense of inner peace
- Deepens meditative experience

7. Zen Meditation (Zazen)

1. Overview
- Zen meditation, or Zazen, is a traditional Buddhist practice that emphasizes seated meditation and mindfulness of the present moment. It often involves observing the breath and sitting in a specific posture.

2. Techniques
- Posture: Sit on a cushion (zafu) with legs crossed or in a kneeling position, keeping the spine straight and hands in a specific mudra (hand position).
- Breath Observation: Focus on the breath as it naturally flows in and out. Count breaths if helpful, starting over after reaching ten.
- Koan Practice: Some Zen practitioners use koans (paradoxical questions or statements) to deepen their meditation and insight.

3. Benefits
- Enhances mindfulness and presence
- Promotes mental clarity and insight
- Reduces stress and anxiety
- Deepens spiritual practice

Conclusion

Exploring different meditation styles allows you to find practices that resonate with you and meet your specific needs. Each style offers unique techniques and benefits, providing various ways to deepen your meditation practice. By experimenting with mindfulness meditation, loving-kindness meditation, body scan meditation, visualization meditation, breath-focused meditation, mantra meditation, and Zen meditation, you can discover the approaches that best support your journey toward greater mindfulness, relaxation, and self-awareness. As you continue to explore and integrate these styles into your routine, you will likely find that your meditation practice becomes more enriching and transformative.

Incorporating Mantras

Mantra meditation is a powerful and ancient practice that involves the repetition of specific words, phrases, or sounds to aid concentration, deepen meditation, and promote a sense of inner peace and clarity. Incorporating mantras into your meditation practice can enhance your focus, elevate your spiritual practice, and help you achieve a deeper state of relaxation and mindfulness. This section explores the concept of mantras, how to choose one, and practical tips for integrating mantras into your meditation routine.

Understanding Mantras

1. Definition of Mantra
- A mantra is a word, phrase, or sound that is repeated during meditation. The term "mantra" comes from the Sanskrit words "manas" (mind) and "tra" (tool), meaning a tool for the mind. Mantras are used to focus the mind and cultivate a deeper state of meditation.

2. Origins and Traditions
- Mantras have their origins in various spiritual traditions, including Hinduism, Buddhism, and Jainism. They are often chanted in languages such as Sanskrit, Pali, or Tibetan and hold spiritual significance and

vibrational power.

3. Purpose of Mantras

- Mantras serve several purposes, including calming the mind, enhancing concentration, invoking spiritual energies, and connecting with a higher consciousness. The repetition of mantras can create a meditative rhythm that helps transcend ordinary thoughts and distractions.

Choosing a Mantra

1. Personal Resonance

- Select a mantra that resonates with you personally. It could be a word or phrase that holds special meaning, inspires you, or brings a sense of peace and comfort. The mantra should feel right and align with your intentions and goals for meditation.

2. Traditional Mantras

- Many practitioners choose traditional mantras that have been used for centuries. Some popular traditional mantras include:

- Om: A universal sound representing the essence of the universe and the interconnectedness of all things.

- Om Mani Padme Hum: A Tibetan Buddhist mantra invoking compassion and wisdom.

- So Hum: A Sanskrit mantra meaning "I am that," reflecting the unity of individual and universal consciousness.

3. Affirmations

- You can also create your own mantras in the form of positive affirmations. Examples include:

- "I am calm and centered."
- "Peace begins with me."
- "I am open to love and compassion."

Techniques for Mantra Meditation

1. Silent Repetition

- Sit comfortably with your spine straight and eyes closed. Begin by taking a few deep breaths to relax. Silently repeat your chosen mantra in your mind, synchronizing it with your breath if desired. Focus on the sound and vibration of the mantra, gently bringing your mind back to it whenever it wanders.

2. Chanting Aloud

- Chanting mantras aloud can amplify their vibrational effects. Sit comfortably and take a few deep breaths. Begin chanting your mantra aloud in a steady, rhythmic manner. Feel the vibrations in your body and listen to the sound of your voice. This technique can be particularly powerful in group settings.

3. Mala Beads

- Mala beads are a traditional tool used to count mantra repetitions. A mala typically consists of 108 beads. Hold the mala in your hand and use your thumb to move from one bead to the next with each repetition of the mantra. This tactile method can enhance focus and keep track of repetitions.

4. Breath Integration

- Integrate your mantra with your breath to deepen the meditative experience. For example, silently repeat "So" on the inhalation and

"Hum" on the exhalation. This synchronization helps maintain a steady rhythm and anchors your attention to both the breath and the mantra.

Benefits of Mantra Meditation

1. Enhanced Concentration

- Repeating a mantra helps to anchor your mind, reducing distractions and enhancing concentration. This focused attention can lead to a deeper and more immersive meditation experience.

2. Stress Reduction

- The rhythmic repetition of a mantra induces a state of relaxation and calm. It can lower stress levels, reduce anxiety, and promote a sense of inner peace and well-being.

3. Spiritual Connection

- Many mantras have spiritual significance and are believed to carry vibrational energy. Repeating these mantras can help you connect with your spiritual self and cultivate a sense of unity with the universe.

4. Emotional Healing

- Mantra meditation can facilitate emotional healing by bringing subconscious thoughts and feelings to the surface. The soothing repetition of a mantra provides comfort and helps process and release emotional blockages.

Practical Tips for Incorporating Mantras

1. Start with Short Sessions

- If you are new to mantra meditation, start with short sessions of 5-10 minutes. Gradually increase the duration as you become more comfortable with the practice.

2. Create a Routine

- Incorporate mantra meditation into your daily routine. Consistency is key to reaping the benefits of the practice. Choose a regular time and place for your meditation sessions to establish a habit.

3. Combine with Other Practices

- Mantra meditation can be combined with other forms of meditation, such as mindfulness or loving-kindness meditation. Experiment with different combinations to find what works best for you.

4. Stay Patient and Persistent

- Like any meditation practice, mantra meditation requires patience and persistence. It's normal for the mind to wander. Gently bring your focus back to the mantra each time this happens, without judgment.

5. Seek Guidance if Needed

- If you're unsure about which mantra to choose or how to practice, seek guidance from experienced practitioners or meditation teachers. They can provide valuable insights and support to help you deepen your practice.

Conclusion

Incorporating mantras into your meditation practice can significantly enhance your focus, relaxation, and spiritual connection. By choosing a mantra that resonates with you and practicing it regularly, you can deepen your meditation experience and cultivate a greater sense of peace and clarity. Whether you prefer silent repetition, chanting aloud, or using mala beads, mantra meditation offers a versatile and powerful tool to support your mindfulness journey. As you explore and integrate mantras into your practice, you will discover their profound ability to transform your meditation and enrich your life.

Guided Meditations for Specific Goals

Guided meditations can be tailored to meet specific goals and address particular needs, providing targeted benefits and enhancing your overall well-being. Whether you are looking to reduce stress, improve focus, enhance sleep, or foster emotional healing, there are guided meditations designed to help you achieve these outcomes. This section explores various guided meditations for specific goals and offers practical advice on how to incorporate them into your practice.

1. Stress Relief

1. Overview

   - Stress relief meditations are designed to help you relax, release tension, and cultivate a sense of calm. These meditations often focus on breathing techniques, progressive relaxation, and visualization to soothe the nervous system.

2. Techniques

- Deep Breathing: Guided instructions on diaphragmatic breathing to reduce stress and promote relaxation.

- Progressive Muscle Relaxation: A technique that involves tensing and then relaxing different muscle groups to release physical tension.

- Calming Visualization: Visualizing serene and peaceful scenes, such as a beach or forest, to create a sense of tranquility.

3. Recommended Resources

- Apps: Calm, Headspace, Insight Timer
- YouTube Channels: The Honest Guys, Michael Sealey
- Books: "The Relaxation Response" by Herbert Benson

2. Improved Focus and Concentration

1. Overview

- Meditations for focus and concentration are designed to enhance your ability to stay present and attentive. These sessions often involve mindfulness practices and techniques to sharpen mental clarity.

2. Techniques

- Mindful Breathing: Focusing on the breath to anchor your attention and improve concentration.

- Counting Breath: Counting each breath cycle to maintain focus and reduce distractions.

- Body Scan: Scanning the body for sensations to stay grounded in the present moment.

3. Recommended Resources

- Apps: Focus@Will, Headspace, Insight Timer

- YouTube Channels: Yoga with Adriene, Tara Brach
- Books: "The Mindful Athlete" by George Mumford

3. Better Sleep

1. Overview
- Guided meditations for sleep are designed to help you unwind, relax, and prepare your mind and body for restful sleep. These meditations typically include calming visualizations, body scans, and sleep-inducing affirmations.

2. Techniques
- Body Scan for Sleep: Progressive relaxation from head to toe to release tension and promote sleep.
- Sleep Stories: Narratives designed to soothe the mind and lull you into sleep.
- Nighttime Affirmations: Positive statements to ease the mind and encourage restful sleep.

3. Recommended Resources
- Apps: Calm, Sleep Cycle, Insight Timer
- YouTube Channels: The Honest Guys, Jason Stephenson
- Books: "The Sleep Solution" by W. Chris Winter

4. Emotional Healing and Self-Compassion

1. Overview
- Meditations for emotional healing and self-compassion focus on cultivating kindness, compassion, and acceptance towards oneself.

These practices help to heal emotional wounds and foster a positive self-image.

2. Techniques

- Loving-Kindness Meditation: Generating feelings of compassion and love towards oneself and others.
- Self-Compassion Exercises: Guided practices that encourage self-kindness and acceptance.
- Healing Visualization: Visualizing healing light or scenarios to promote emotional well-being.

3. Recommended Resources

- Apps: Calm, Insight Timer, MyLife Meditation
- YouTube Channels: Kristin Neff, Tara Brach
- Books: "Radical Acceptance" by Tara Brach, "Self-Compassion" by Kristin Neff

5. Creativity and Problem-Solving

1. Overview

- Meditations to boost creativity and problem-solving abilities often involve visualization, free-form thinking, and exercises that encourage the flow of creative ideas.

2. Techniques

- Creative Visualization: Imagining creative scenarios or solutions to stimulate creativity.
- Mind Mapping Meditation: Using meditation to explore ideas and connections in a relaxed state.
- Open Awareness: Allowing the mind to flow freely and observe

thoughts without judgment to encourage creative insights.

3. Recommended Resources
  - Apps: Headspace, Insight Timer, Brain.fm
  - YouTube Channels: Jason Stephenson, Michael Sealey
  - Books: "The Artist's Way" by Julia Cameron

6. Pain Management

1. Overview
- Guided meditations for pain management focus on altering the perception of pain and promoting relaxation and healing. These meditations can help reduce the intensity of pain and improve the quality of life.

2. Techniques
- Body Scan for Pain Relief: Focusing on different body parts to reduce pain and tension.
- Breath Awareness: Using the breath to create a sense of calm and alleviate pain.
- Healing Visualization: Imagining healing light or energy flowing through the body to relieve pain.

3. Recommended Resources
  - Apps: Calm, Insight Timer, MyPainAway
  - YouTube Channels: The Honest Guys, Michael Sealey
  - Books: "You Are Not Your Pain" by Vidyamala Burch and Danny Penman

7. Spiritual Growth and Connection

1. Overview
- Meditations for spiritual growth aim to deepen your connection with your higher self, the universe, or a higher power. These practices often involve elements of contemplation, gratitude, and spiritual inquiry.

2. Techniques
- Contemplative Meditation: Reflecting on spiritual questions or teachings to gain deeper insights.
- Gratitude Meditation: Focusing on feelings of gratitude to enhance spiritual awareness.
- Connecting with Higher Self: Visualizations and affirmations to strengthen your spiritual connection.

3. Recommended Resources
- Apps: Insight Timer, Calm, Headspace
- YouTube Channels: Deepak Chopra, Eckhart Tolle
- Books: "The Power of Now" by Eckhart Tolle, "The Seat of the Soul" by Gary Zukav

Conclusion

Guided meditations tailored to specific goals can significantly enhance your meditation practice by addressing your unique needs and aspirations. Whether you aim to reduce stress, improve focus, enhance sleep, foster emotional healing, boost creativity, manage pain, or deepen your spiritual connection, there are guided meditations available to support you. By incorporating these targeted meditations into your routine, you can experience more profound and specific benefits, leading to a more fulfilling and balanced life. As you explore different guided meditations, remember to choose those that resonate with you and align with your personal goals, allowing you to make the most of your meditation practice.

5

Overcoming Common Challenges

Dealing with Distractions

Distractions are a common obstacle in meditation practice, particularly for beginners. Learning to manage and minimize distractions can enhance your meditation experience and help you maintain focus and achieve deeper states of relaxation and mindfulness. This section explores strategies for dealing with both internal and external distractions during meditation.

Understanding Distractions

1. Internal Distractions

   - Internal distractions come from within your mind and body. They include thoughts, emotions, physical sensations, and mental chatter. These distractions can be particularly challenging as they are intrinsic to your personal experience.

2. External Distractions

- External distractions are environmental factors that disrupt your focus. These can include noise, interruptions, uncomfortable surroundings, or other sensory disturbances. Creating a conducive environment can help mitigate these distractions.

Strategies for Managing Internal Distractions

1. Acknowledge and Accept

- The first step in dealing with internal distractions is to acknowledge and accept them without judgment. Recognize that it is natural for the mind to wander and that distractions are a normal part of the meditation process.

2. Return to Your Focus

- Whenever you notice your mind wandering, gently bring your attention back to your chosen point of focus, such as your breath, a mantra, or a guided instruction. This practice of returning helps strengthen your concentration over time.

3. Label Your Thoughts

- If you find yourself caught in a stream of thoughts, try labeling them (e.g., "thinking," "worrying," "planning"). This labeling can create a sense of detachment and make it easier to let go of the distraction and return to your meditation.

4. Use a Mantra

- Incorporating a mantra into your meditation can help anchor your mind and reduce internal distractions. Repeating a soothing word or phrase can provide a focal point that draws your attention away from distracting thoughts.

5. Practice Mindfulness

- Develop a mindful attitude towards distractions. Instead of fighting them, observe them with curiosity and openness. Notice the nature of the distraction and how it affects you, then gently refocus on your meditation.

6. Body Scan

- Conduct a brief body scan to identify and release physical tension that might be causing distractions. Bringing awareness to different parts of your body can help you relax and minimize physical discomfort.

Strategies for Managing External Distractions

1. Create a Conducive Environment

- Choose a quiet and comfortable space for meditation where you are less likely to be disturbed. Inform household members of your meditation time to minimize interruptions.

2. Use Noise-Canceling Headphones

- If you are in a noisy environment, consider using noise-canceling headphones or earplugs to block out external sounds. Alternatively, you can play soft, ambient music or nature sounds to mask background noise.

3. Set Boundaries

- Establish boundaries to prevent interruptions during your meditation. Put your phone on silent or airplane mode, and place a "do not disturb" sign on your door if necessary.

4. Comfortable Seating

- Ensure that you are seated comfortably to avoid physical discomfort that can distract you. Use cushions, blankets, or a comfortable chair to support your posture.

5. Adapt to the Environment

- Accept that some level of external noise and activity is inevitable. Instead of resisting these distractions, try to integrate them into your practice. Use them as an opportunity to strengthen your focus and deepen your mindfulness.

Practical Exercises for Dealing with Distractions

1. Mindful Breathing Exercise

- Sit comfortably and close your eyes. Focus on your breath as it flows in and out. If a distraction arises, gently acknowledge it and return your attention to your breath. Repeat this process each time you notice your mind wandering.

2. Counting Breaths

- Count each breath cycle (inhale and exhale) up to ten, then start over. If you lose count due to a distraction, start again from one. This practice helps maintain focus and minimizes the impact of distractions.

3. Visualization

- Use visualization to create a mental image of a peaceful place. Focus on the details of this place, such as the colors, sounds, and sensations. If distractions arise, gently guide your attention back to your visualization.

4. Guided Meditation

- Follow a guided meditation that specifically addresses dealing with distractions. The guide can provide instructions and reminders to help you stay focused and manage interruptions.

Long-Term Strategies for Reducing Distractions

1. Regular Practice

- Consistency is key to reducing distractions over time. The more regularly you meditate, the better you become at managing distractions and maintaining focus.

2. Mindfulness in Daily Life

- Incorporate mindfulness into your daily activities. Practicing mindfulness throughout the day can enhance your ability to stay present and focused during meditation.

3. Reduce Overall Stress

- Addressing sources of stress in your life can reduce internal distractions. Engage in stress-reducing activities such as exercise, hobbies, or spending time in nature to create a more relaxed state of mind.

4. Healthy Lifestyle

- Maintain a healthy lifestyle by eating well, staying hydrated, and getting enough sleep. Physical well-being can significantly impact your mental clarity and ability to focus.

Conclusion

Dealing with distractions is a common challenge in meditation practice, but with the right strategies, you can learn to manage and minimize them effectively. By creating a conducive environment, practicing mindfulness, and using specific techniques to refocus your attention, you can enhance your ability to stay present and deepen your meditation experience. Remember that distractions are a natural part of the process, and with patience and persistence, you can overcome them and achieve a more focused and fulfilling meditation practice.

Managing Restlessness and Anxiety

Restlessness and anxiety are common experiences during meditation, especially for beginners. These feelings can make it challenging to maintain focus and achieve a state of calm. However, with the right strategies, you can learn to manage restlessness and anxiety effectively, allowing you to deepen your meditation practice. This section explores practical techniques to help you address and overcome these challenges.

Understanding Restlessness and Anxiety

1. Restlessness

 - Restlessness often manifests as a sense of physical or mental agitation. It can be driven by an inability to sit still, racing thoughts, or a constant urge to move. Recognizing restlessness as a natural response can help you approach it with greater patience and understanding.

2. Anxiety

- Anxiety during meditation can arise from various sources, including stress, worries about the future, or past experiences. It may present as a tightness in the chest, rapid heartbeat, or a feeling of unease. Understanding that anxiety is a common and manageable part of meditation can help you navigate it more effectively.

Strategies for Managing Restlessness

1. Physical Adjustments

- Comfortable Posture: Ensure you are seated comfortably. Use cushions, blankets, or a chair to support your posture and reduce physical discomfort.

- Movement Breaks: If restlessness becomes overwhelming, allow yourself short breaks to stretch or move gently. Returning to meditation after addressing physical needs can help you settle more easily.

2. Focused Attention

- Breath Awareness: Direct your attention to your breath. Notice the sensation of the air entering and leaving your nostrils or the rise and fall of your chest or abdomen. Focusing on the breath can anchor your mind and reduce restlessness.

- Body Scan: Conduct a body scan to bring awareness to different parts of your body. This practice can help you identify and release areas of tension, promoting relaxation.

3. Mindful Acceptance

- Observe Without Judgment: Acknowledge restlessness without judgment. Observe the sensations and thoughts associated with it, and remind yourself that it is a temporary experience.

- Non-Resistance: Instead of resisting restlessness, accept it as part of your current experience. Allowing restlessness to be present can reduce its intensity and help it pass more quickly.

4. Engaging the Senses

- Sound Meditation: Focus on ambient sounds or use a sound meditation app to engage your auditory senses. This can help divert your mind from restlessness and bring you back to the present moment.

- Visual Focus: If closing your eyes increases restlessness, try meditating with your eyes open, focusing softly on a point in front of you or a visual object like a candle flame.

Strategies for Managing Anxiety

1. Breath Control

- Deep Breathing: Practice deep, diaphragmatic breathing to calm the nervous system. Inhale deeply through your nose, allowing your abdomen to expand, and exhale slowly through your mouth.

- 4-7-8 Breathing: Inhale for a count of 4, hold for 7, and exhale for 8. This technique can help slow your heart rate and promote relaxation.

2. Grounding Techniques

- Five Senses Exercise: Identify five things you can see, four things you can touch, three things you can hear, two things you can smell, and one thing you can taste. This exercise can ground you in the present moment and reduce anxiety.

- Feet on the Floor: Place both feet firmly on the ground and notice the sensations. This simple grounding technique can help you feel more stable and connected to the present.

3. Guided Imagery

- Safe Place Visualization: Imagine a place where you feel safe and calm. Visualize it in detail, focusing on the sights, sounds, smells, and feelings associated with it. Guided imagery can create a mental escape from anxiety.

- Healing Light Visualization: Visualize a warm, healing light entering your body with each inhale, and spreading calm and relaxation throughout your body with each exhale.

4. Affirmations and Mantras

- Positive Affirmations: Repeat calming affirmations such as "I am safe," "I am calm," or "This too shall pass." Affirmations can help shift your mindset and reduce anxiety.

- Mantra Repetition: Use a calming mantra such as "Om" or "Peace" to focus your mind and create a sense of inner calm.

5. Mindful Observation

- Labeling Emotions: When anxiety arises, label it mentally (e.g., "anxiety," "fear," "worry"). This practice creates a sense of detachment and can reduce the power of anxious thoughts.

- Observe Without Reacting: Observe your anxious thoughts and sensations without reacting to them. Imagine them as clouds passing in the sky, allowing them to come and go without attachment.

Long-Term Strategies for Reducing Restlessness and Anxiety

1. Consistent Practice

- Regular meditation practice can help reduce overall levels of restlessness and anxiety. Consistency builds familiarity and comfort with the meditation process, making it easier to manage these challenges.

2. Lifestyle Adjustments

- Addressing lifestyle factors such as diet, exercise, and sleep can have a significant impact on your ability to manage restlessness and anxiety. A healthy lifestyle supports a calm and balanced mind.

3. Mindfulness in Daily Life

- Incorporate mindfulness into your daily activities. Practicing mindfulness throughout the day can enhance your ability to stay present and reduce anxiety during meditation.

4. Professional Support

- If anxiety or restlessness persists and significantly impacts your well-being, consider seeking support from a mental health professional. Therapy, counseling, or mindfulness-based stress reduction programs can provide additional tools and support.

Conclusion

Managing restlessness and anxiety during meditation is a common challenge, but with the right strategies, you can learn to navigate these experiences effectively. By incorporating techniques such as breath control, grounding exercises, guided imagery, and mindful observation, you can reduce the impact of restlessness and anxiety on your practice. Consistent meditation, lifestyle adjustments, and mindfulness in daily life can further support your ability to stay calm and focused. Remember that both restlessness and anxiety are natural parts of the meditation journey, and with patience and persistence, you can overcome these obstacles and deepen your practice.

Consistency and Discipline

Maintaining a consistent meditation practice requires discipline and dedication. Many beginners face challenges in making meditation a regular part of their daily routine. This section provides strategies and tips to help you build consistency and discipline in your meditation practice, ensuring that you can reap the full benefits of regular meditation.

The Importance of Consistency and Discipline

1. Maximizes Benefits

- Regular meditation practice is essential for experiencing the full range of benefits, including reduced stress, improved focus, enhanced emotional well-being, and greater self-awareness. Consistency helps to solidify these benefits over time.

2. Builds Habit

- Consistency is key to forming a habit. By making meditation a regular part of your daily routine, it becomes a natural and integral part of your life, requiring less effort and willpower over time.

3. Deepens Practice

- A consistent practice allows for gradual deepening and refinement of your meditation skills. Regular practice helps you move beyond surface-level experiences and achieve deeper states of mindfulness and relaxation.

Strategies for Building Consistency and Discipline

1. Set Clear Intentions and Goals

- Define Your Purpose: Clearly articulate why you want to meditate. Understanding your motivations can help you stay committed to your practice.

- Set Specific Goals: Establish realistic and specific goals for your meditation practice, such as meditating for a certain number of minutes each day or completing a particular number of sessions each week.

2. Create a Routine

- Choose a Regular Time: Select a specific time of day for your meditation practice. Morning and evening are popular choices, but the best time is the one that fits seamlessly into your daily schedule.

- Establish a Ritual: Develop a pre-meditation ritual to signal to your mind and body that it's time to meditate. This could include activities like lighting a candle, playing soft music, or performing a few stretches.

3. Start Small and Gradual

- Begin with Short Sessions: Start with shorter meditation sessions (5-10 minutes) and gradually increase the duration as you become more comfortable. This approach helps prevent feelings of overwhelm and builds confidence.

- Incremental Progress: Gradually extend the length of your meditation sessions and increase the frequency. Small, incremental progress is more sustainable and less daunting.

4. Use Reminders and Tools

- Set Alarms and Reminders: Use alarms, reminders, or calendar notifications to prompt you to meditate at your chosen time. Consistent reminders can help establish and maintain your routine.

- Meditation Apps: Utilize meditation apps that offer guided sessions, progress tracking, and reminders. Apps like Headspace, Calm, and Insight Timer provide structure and support for building consistency.

5. Create a Dedicated Space

- Designate a Meditation Area: Set up a specific space in your home for meditation. This space should be quiet, comfortable, and free from distractions. Having a dedicated area can reinforce the habit and make it easier to start each session.

- Personalize Your Space: Add items that enhance your meditation experience, such as cushions, blankets, candles, or calming artwork. A pleasant environment can increase your motivation to meditate regularly.

6. Track Your Progress

- Maintain a Meditation Journal: Keep a journal to record your meditation sessions, noting the date, duration, and any insights or experiences. Tracking your progress can provide motivation and a sense of accomplishment.

- Use Apps with Tracking Features: Many meditation apps offer tracking features that log your sessions and provide feedback on your consistency and progress.

Overcoming Obstacles to Consistency

1. Addressing Lack of Time

- Prioritize Meditation: Treat meditation as a non-negotiable part of your day, similar to eating or sleeping. Prioritizing your practice ensures it becomes an integral part of your routine.

- Incorporate into Daily Activities: Integrate mindfulness into everyday activities, such as mindful walking, eating, or commuting. Even short, informal practices can reinforce the habit.

2. Dealing with Resistance

- Acknowledge Resistance: Recognize that resistance is a normal part of building any new habit. Acknowledge it without judgment and remind yourself of the benefits and reasons for your practice.

- Use Positive Reinforcement: Reward yourself for maintaining your practice. Positive reinforcement can increase motivation and make the habit more enjoyable.

3. Managing Boredom

- Vary Your Practice: Introduce variety into your meditation practice by exploring different styles and techniques. This can keep your practice interesting and prevent boredom.

- Stay Curious: Approach each session with curiosity, even if it feels repetitive. Each meditation session is unique, and staying open to new experiences can enhance your practice.

4. Finding Support and Accountability

- Join a Meditation Group: Joining a meditation group or class can provide support, encouragement, and accountability. Practicing with others can enhance motivation and commitment.

- Share Your Goals: Share your meditation goals with a friend or family member who can offer support and check in on your progress.

Long-Term Strategies for Sustaining Disciplineeflect on the Benefits

1.- Regularly reflect on the benefits you've experienced from meditation. This can reinforce your commitment and remind you of the positive impact on your well-being.

2. Continue Learning

- Stay engaged by continuing to learn about meditation through books, workshops, and courses. Deepening your knowledge can inspire and motivate you to maintain your practice.

3. Embrace Flexibility

- Be flexible with your practice. Life circumstances may change, and it's important to adapt your meditation routine accordingly. Flexibility ensures that meditation remains a sustainable and enjoyable part of your life.

4. Cultivate Self-Compassion

- Approach your meditation practice with self-compassion. Recognize that building a consistent practice takes time and that it's okay to miss a session occasionally. Compassionate self-acceptance fosters a positive relationship with your practice.

Conclusion

Consistency and discipline are crucial for establishing and maintaining a regular meditation practice. By setting clear goals, creating a routine, starting small, using reminders, and tracking your progress, you can build a sustainable meditation habit. Overcoming obstacles such as lack of time, resistance, boredom, and finding support can further enhance your ability to stay committed. With patience, persistence, and self-compassion, you can develop a consistent and disciplined meditation practice that brings lasting benefits to your mind, body, and spirit.

6

The Science Behind Meditation

How Meditation Affects the Brain

Meditation has long been practiced for its mental, emotional, and spiritual benefits. In recent decades, scientific research has begun to uncover the physiological changes that occur in the brain as a result of regular meditation practice. This section explores the ways in which meditation affects the brain, enhancing our understanding of its profound impact on cognitive function, emotional regulation, and overall mental health.

Neuroplasticity and Meditation

1. Definition of Neuroplasticity

- Neuroplasticity refers to the brain's ability to reorganize itself by forming new neural connections throughout life. This adaptability allows the brain to recover from injuries, adapt to new situations, and improve cognitive functions through learning and experience.

2. Impact of Meditation on Neuroplasticity

- Regular meditation practice enhances neuroplasticity, promoting positive changes in brain structure and function. This increased plasticity is associated with improved learning, memory, and emotional regulation.

Changes in Brain Structure

1. Increased Gray Matter

- Hippocampus: Studies have shown that meditation increases gray matter density in the hippocampus, a region associated with learning, memory, and emotional regulation. This growth supports enhanced cognitive functions and emotional resilience.

- Prefrontal Cortex: Meditation also increases gray matter in the prefrontal cortex, which is involved in executive functions such as decision-making, attention, and self-control. This enhancement leads to better focus, planning, and emotional regulation.

2. Reduced Amygdala Size

- The amygdala is the brain's fear center, responsible for processing emotions such as stress and anxiety. Meditation has been shown to reduce the size and activity of the amygdala, leading to decreased emotional reactivity and lower levels of stress and anxiety.

Functional Changes in the Brain

1. Enhanced Connectivity

- Default Mode Network (DMN): The DMN is a network of brain regions involved in self-referential thinking and mind-wandering.

Meditation reduces activity in the DMN, leading to decreased rumination and increased present-moment awareness.

- Attention Networks: Meditation strengthens the connectivity within attention networks, improving the brain's ability to focus and maintain attention. This enhanced connectivity supports better cognitive performance and task management.

2. Improved Emotional Regulation

- Anterior Cingulate Cortex (ACC): The ACC plays a key role in regulating emotions and impulses. Meditation increases activity in the ACC, enhancing emotional regulation and reducing impulsivity.

- Insula: The insula is involved in body awareness and emotional processing. Meditation increases insula activity, improving interoception (awareness of internal body states) and emotional awareness.

Neurochemical Changes

1. Increased Production of Neurotransmitters

- Serotonin: Meditation increases serotonin levels, a neurotransmitter associated with mood regulation, happiness, and overall well-being. Higher serotonin levels contribute to improved mood and reduced symptoms of depression.

- GABA: Gamma-aminobutyric acid (GABA) is a neurotransmitter that inhibits neural activity, promoting relaxation and reducing anxiety. Meditation increases GABA levels, supporting a calm and relaxed state.

2. Reduced Cortisol Levels

- Cortisol is a stress hormone that, when chronically elevated, can have detrimental effects on health. Meditation has been shown to reduce cortisol levels, leading to decreased stress and improved overall health.

Cognitive Benefits

1. Improved Attention and Concentration

- Meditation enhances the brain's attention networks, leading to better focus, concentration, and sustained attention. These improvements are particularly beneficial for tasks that require prolonged mental effort and precision.

2. Enhanced Memory and Learning

- The increase in gray matter density in the hippocampus supports improved memory and learning capabilities. Regular meditation practice enhances both short-term and long-term memory, aiding in information retention and recall.

3. Greater Cognitive Flexibility

- Meditation improves cognitive flexibility, the ability to switch between different tasks or thoughts efficiently. This flexibility supports better problem-solving skills and adaptive thinking.

Emotional and Psychological Benefits

1. Reduced Anxiety and Depression

- The changes in brain structure and function associated with meditation lead to reduced symptoms of anxiety and depression. The decreased size and activity of the amygdala, along with increased serotonin production, contribute to improved emotional well-being.

2. Increased Resilience to Stress

- Meditation enhances the brain's ability to regulate stress responses, making practitioners more resilient to stressors. The reduction in cortisol levels and increased activity in regions responsible for emotional regulation support this resilience.

3. Enhanced Emotional Intelligence

- By improving interoception and emotional awareness, meditation enhances emotional intelligence. Practitioners become more attuned to their emotions and better able to manage them, leading to improved interpersonal relationships and self-awareness.

Conclusion

Meditation induces profound changes in the brain, promoting neuroplasticity, altering brain structure, and enhancing brain function. These changes result in numerous cognitive, emotional, and psychological benefits, including improved attention, memory, emotional regulation, and stress resilience. Understanding how meditation affects the brain underscores the importance of incorporating this practice into daily life. By regularly engaging in meditation, individuals can harness these benefits to improve their mental health and overall well-being.

Physiological Benefits

Meditation is well-known for its mental and emotional benefits, but it also has profound effects on the physical body. Scientific research has demonstrated that regular meditation practice can lead to various physiological improvements, contributing to overall health and well-being. This section explores the key physiological benefits of meditation, including its impact on the cardiovascular system, immune function, and pain management.

Cardiovascular Health

1. Reduced Blood Pressure
 - Meditation promotes relaxation and reduces stress, which can help lower blood pressure. Studies have shown that mindfulness and transcendental meditation can significantly reduce both systolic and diastolic blood pressure, decreasing the risk of hypertension-related health issues.

2. Improved Heart Rate Variability
 - Heart rate variability (HRV) is a measure of the variation in time between heartbeats. Higher HRV is associated with better cardiovascular health and resilience to stress. Meditation has been shown to increase HRV, indicating improved autonomic nervous system function and enhanced heart health.

3. Decreased Risk of Heart Disease
 - By lowering blood pressure, reducing stress, and improving lipid profiles, meditation can decrease the risk of heart disease. Regular meditation practice is associated with lower levels of LDL cholesterol and triglycerides, contributing to better cardiovascular health.

Enhanced Immune Function

1. Increased Immune Cell Activity

- Meditation has been found to enhance the activity of immune cells, such as natural killer cells and lymphocytes. These cells play a crucial role in defending the body against infections and diseases. Increased immune cell activity improves the body's ability to fight off pathogens and maintain overall health.

2. Reduced Inflammatory Markers

- Chronic inflammation is linked to various diseases, including heart disease, diabetes, and cancer. Meditation reduces the levels of inflammatory markers in the body, such as C-reactive protein (CRP) and interleukin-6 (IL-6). Lower inflammation levels contribute to better immune function and overall health.

3. Improved Antibody Response

- Studies have shown that meditation can enhance the body's antibody response to vaccines. This improved response indicates a stronger and more effective immune system, better prepared to protect against illnesses.

Pain Management

1. Reduced Perception of Pain

- Meditation can alter the way the brain perceives pain, reducing the intensity and unpleasantness of pain sensations. Techniques such as mindfulness meditation and loving-kindness meditation have been shown to decrease pain perception and increase pain tolerance.

2. Enhanced Pain Coping Mechanisms

- Meditation improves emotional regulation and increases resilience, helping individuals cope more effectively with chronic pain. By fostering a non-judgmental awareness of pain, meditation enables practitioners to manage pain without becoming overwhelmed by it.

3. Lower Pain-Related Stress

- Chronic pain often leads to stress and anxiety, which can exacerbate pain symptoms. Meditation reduces stress levels and promotes relaxation, helping to break the cycle of pain and stress and improve overall pain management.

Respiratory Health

1. Improved Breathing Efficiency

- Meditation techniques that focus on breath awareness and control, such as diaphragmatic breathing and alternate nostril breathing, enhance breathing efficiency. These practices strengthen the respiratory muscles, increase lung capacity, and improve oxygen exchange.

2. Reduction in Respiratory Rate

- Regular meditation practice can lead to a lower resting respiratory rate, indicating more efficient and relaxed breathing patterns. A lower respiratory rate is associated with reduced stress and better overall respiratory health.

3. Management of Respiratory Conditions

- Meditation has been shown to help manage symptoms of respiratory conditions such as asthma and chronic obstructive pulmonary disease (COPD). By promoting relaxation and improving lung function, meditation can reduce the severity and frequency of symptoms.

Digestive Health

1. Improved Digestion

- Stress and anxiety can negatively impact digestion, leading to issues such as irritable bowel syndrome (IBS) and indigestion. Meditation promotes relaxation and reduces stress, improving digestive function and alleviating symptoms of digestive disorders.

2. Enhanced Gut-Brain Connection

- The gut-brain axis is a bidirectional communication system between the gut and the brain. Meditation enhances this connection, promoting better digestive health and overall well-being. Improved gut-brain communication can lead to more efficient digestion and reduced gastrointestinal distress.

3. Balanced Microbiome

- Emerging research suggests that meditation may positively influence the gut microbiome, the community of microorganisms living in the digestive tract. A balanced microbiome is crucial for digestive health, immune function, and overall well-being.

Endocrine Health

1. Regulation of Stress Hormones

- Meditation helps regulate the production of stress hormones such as cortisol and adrenaline. Lower levels of these hormones contribute to reduced stress and anxiety, better immune function, and improved overall health.

2. Enhanced Hormonal Balance

- Meditation can promote hormonal balance by reducing stress and improving overall health. Balanced hormone levels are crucial for various bodily functions, including metabolism, reproduction, and mood regulation.

3. Improved Insulin Sensitivity

- Regular meditation practice has been linked to improved insulin sensitivity, which is essential for maintaining healthy blood sugar levels. Better insulin sensitivity can reduce the risk of type 2 diabetes and support overall metabolic health.

Conclusion

Meditation offers a wide range of physiological benefits that contribute to overall health and well-being. From improved cardiovascular health and enhanced immune function to better pain management and respiratory health, regular meditation practice can lead to significant physical improvements. Understanding these physiological benefits underscores the importance of incorporating meditation into your daily routine. By doing so, you can support your body's health and enhance your quality of life.

Psychological Benefits

Meditation is widely recognized for its profound psychological benefits. Scientific research has demonstrated that regular meditation practice can significantly improve mental health, emotional well-being, and overall cognitive function. This section explores the key psychological benefits of meditation, including its impact on stress reduction, emotional regulation, and mental clarity.

Stress Reduction

1. Lower Cortisol Levels

   - Meditation helps to reduce the production of cortisol, the primary stress hormone. Lower cortisol levels lead to decreased physical and mental stress, promoting a sense of calm and relaxation.

2. Activation of the Relaxation Response

   - Meditation activates the body's relaxation response, counteracting the stress response. This activation helps to lower heart rate, reduce blood pressure, and promote a state of deep relaxation and well-being.

3. Enhanced Resilience to Stress

   - Regular meditation practice enhances the brain's ability to manage stress, making individuals more resilient to stressors. This increased resilience helps to prevent stress-related mental health issues, such as anxiety and depression.

Emotional Regulation

1. Increased Emotional Awareness
- Meditation enhances emotional awareness, helping individuals to recognize and understand their emotions more clearly. This heightened awareness allows for better emotional regulation and management.

2. Improved Mood
- Regular meditation practice is associated with improved mood and a greater sense of overall well-being. Meditation increases the production of neurotransmitters such as serotonin and dopamine, which are linked to feelings of happiness and contentment.

3. Reduction in Negative Emotions
- Meditation helps to reduce negative emotions, such as anger, fear, and sadness. By promoting a non-judgmental awareness of thoughts and feelings, meditation allows individuals to process and release negative emotions more effectively.

Mental Clarity and Focus

1. Enhanced Attention and Concentration
- Meditation improves attention and concentration by training the brain to focus on the present moment. This enhanced focus can lead to better performance in tasks that require sustained attention and mental effort.

2. Improved Cognitive Function
- Regular meditation practice has been shown to improve various

aspects of cognitive function, including memory, problem-solving skills, and decision-making. These cognitive benefits are linked to changes in brain structure and function associated with meditation.

3. Greater Mental Flexibility

- Meditation enhances mental flexibility, the ability to adapt to new situations and switch between different tasks or thoughts efficiently. This flexibility supports better problem-solving and adaptive thinking.

Reduced Anxiety and Depression

1. Decreased Symptoms of Anxiety

- Meditation has been shown to reduce symptoms of anxiety, including generalized anxiety disorder (GAD), social anxiety, and panic attacks. By promoting relaxation and reducing stress, meditation helps to alleviate anxiety and its associated symptoms.

2. Reduction in Depressive Symptoms

- Regular meditation practice is effective in reducing symptoms of depression. Meditation helps to increase positive emotions, improve mood, and reduce the severity of depressive episodes.

3. Improved Emotional Resilience

- Meditation enhances emotional resilience, helping individuals to cope more effectively with life's challenges and setbacks. This increased resilience can prevent the onset of anxiety and depression and support long-term mental health.

Enhanced Self-Awareness and Self-Acceptance

1. Increased Self-Awareness

- Meditation promotes self-awareness by encouraging individuals to observe their thoughts, feelings, and behaviors without judgment. This increased awareness can lead to greater self-understanding and personal growth.

2. Greater Self-Acceptance

- Meditation fosters self-acceptance by promoting a non-judgmental attitude towards oneself. This acceptance helps individuals to develop a more positive self-image and a greater sense of self-worth.

3. Improved Interpersonal Relationships

- Enhanced self-awareness and self-acceptance can lead to improved interpersonal relationships. By understanding and accepting themselves, individuals are better able to understand and accept others, leading to more harmonious and fulfilling relationships.

Mindfulness and Present-Moment Awareness

1. Enhanced Mindfulness

- Meditation promotes mindfulness, the practice of being fully present and engaged in the current moment. This enhanced mindfulness can improve overall well-being and lead to a greater sense of fulfillment in daily life.

2. Reduction in Mind-Wandering

- Regular meditation practice reduces mind-wandering, the tendency for the mind to drift away from the present moment. By promoting focused attention, meditation helps individuals to stay present and engaged.

3. Increased Enjoyment of Life

- Mindfulness and present-moment awareness can lead to a greater enjoyment of life. By fully experiencing each moment, individuals can develop a deeper appreciation for the simple pleasures of life.

Spiritual Growth and Connection

1. Enhanced Spiritual Awareness

- For those who practice meditation for spiritual purposes, meditation can enhance spiritual awareness and connection. This increased awareness can lead to a deeper sense of purpose and meaning in life.

2. Greater Sense of Connection

- Meditation can foster a sense of connection to something greater than oneself, whether it is a higher power, the universe, or the interconnectedness of all living beings. This sense of connection can provide comfort, inspiration, and a sense of belonging.

3. Deepened Compassion and Empathy

- Meditation practices such as loving-kindness meditation can enhance feelings of compassion and empathy towards oneself and others. This increased compassion can lead to more harmonious relationships and a greater sense of community.

Conclusion

The psychological benefits of meditation are vast and well-documented. From reducing stress and anxiety to enhancing emotional regulation and cognitive function, meditation offers a powerful tool for improving mental health and overall well-being. By promoting mindfulness, self-awareness, and emotional resilience, regular meditation practice can lead to profound psychological transformation and a greater sense of peace and fulfillment in life. Understanding these benefits underscores the importance of incorporating meditation into daily life to support mental and emotional health.

7

Advanced Techniques and Practices

Chakra Meditation

Chakra meditation is an advanced practice that focuses on the body's energy centers, known as chakras. This form of meditation aims to balance and align these energy centers to promote physical, emotional, and spiritual well-being. This section explores the concept of chakras, the benefits of chakra meditation, and practical techniques to incorporate chakra meditation into your practice.

Understanding Chakras

1. Definition of Chakras

- Chakras are energy centers within the body, originating from ancient Indian spiritual traditions. The word "chakra" means "wheel" or "disk" in Sanskrit, symbolizing the spinning energy at each chakra point. There are seven main chakras aligned along the spine, from the

113

base to the crown of the head.

2. The Seven Main Chakras

- Root Chakra (Muladhara): Located at the base of the spine, associated with survival, stability, and grounding. Its color is red.

- Sacral Chakra (Svadhisthana): Located below the navel, associated with creativity, sexuality, and emotions. Its color is orange.

- Solar Plexus Chakra (Manipura): Located above the navel, associated with personal power, confidence, and willpower. Its color is yellow.

- Heart Chakra (Anahata): Located at the center of the chest, associated with love, compassion, and connection. Its color is green.

- Throat Chakra (Vishuddha): Located at the throat, associated with communication, expression, and truth. Its color is blue.

- Third Eye Chakra (Ajna): Located between the eyebrows, associated with intuition, insight, and wisdom. Its color is indigo.

- Crown Chakra (Sahasrara): Located at the top of the head, associated with spiritual connection and enlightenment. Its color is violet or white.

Benefits of Chakra Meditation

1. Balanced Energy

- Chakra meditation helps balance the energy flow within the body, ensuring that each chakra is neither overactive nor underactive. Balanced chakras contribute to overall physical and emotional well-being.

2. Enhanced Physical Health

- By promoting the free flow of energy, chakra meditation can help alleviate physical ailments associated with blocked or imbalanced chakras. Each chakra corresponds to specific organs and body functions, so balanced chakras can lead to improved health.

3. Emotional and Mental Clarity

- Balancing the chakras can lead to emotional stability and mental clarity. It helps release negative emotions, reduce stress, and promote a positive mindset.

4. Spiritual Growth

- Chakra meditation deepens spiritual awareness and fosters a connection to higher consciousness. It can enhance intuition, insight, and a sense of oneness with the universe.

Techniques for Chakra Meditation

1. Preparation

- Find a quiet and comfortable space where you won't be disturbed. Sit or lie down in a relaxed position with your spine straight. Close your eyes and take a few deep breaths to center yourself.

2. Guided Visualization

- Use guided meditations specifically designed for chakra balancing. These meditations will guide you through visualizing each chakra, often incorporating colors, symbols, and affirmations.

3. Focus on Each Chakra

- Starting from the root chakra, bring your awareness to each chakra in turn. Visualize its associated color and imagine a spinning wheel of energy at each point. Spend a few minutes focusing on each chakra, from the base of the spine to the crown of the head.

4. Chanting and Mantras

- Each chakra has a specific seed sound (bija mantra) that can be chanted to stimulate and balance the energy. Chant the following mantras for each chakra:
    - Root Chakra: "LAM"
    - Sacral Chakra: "VAM"
    - Solar Plexus Chakra: "RAM"
    - Heart Chakra: "YAM"
    - Throat Chakra: "HAM"
    - Third Eye Chakra: "OM" or "AUM"
    - Crown Chakra: Silence or "OM"

5. Breathing Techniques

- Use specific breathing techniques to enhance chakra meditation. Deep, rhythmic breathing can help activate and balance the chakras. For example, you can use alternate nostril breathing to balance the overall energy flow before focusing on individual chakras.

6. Affirmations

- Repeat positive affirmations associated with each chakra to reinforce the balancing process. For example:
    - Root Chakra: "I am grounded and secure."
    - Sacral Chakra: "I am creative and joyful."
    - Solar Plexus Chakra: "I am confident and strong."
    - Heart Chakra: "I am loving and compassionate."
    - Throat Chakra: "I speak my truth with clarity."
    - Third Eye Chakra: "I trust my intuition."
    - Crown Chakra: "I am connected to the divine."

7. Crystal Healing

- Incorporate crystals associated with each chakra to enhance the meditation. Place the corresponding crystal on or near each chakra point during meditation. For example:
  - Root Chakra: Red Jasper or Hematite
  - Sacral Chakra: Carnelian or Orange Calcite
  - Solar Plexus Chakra: Citrine or Yellow Jasper
  - Heart Chakra: Rose Quartz or Green Aventurine
  - Throat Chakra: Blue Lace Agate or Lapis Lazuli
  - Third Eye Chakra: Amethyst or Sodalite
  - Crown Chakra: Clear Quartz or Amethyst

Integrating Chakra Meditation into Your Practice

1. Regular Practice

- Incorporate chakra meditation into your regular meditation routine. Consistent practice is key to maintaining balanced and aligned chakras.

2. Combine with Other Practices

- Combine chakra meditation with other practices such as yoga, breathwork, or mindfulness to enhance its benefits. Yoga poses that align with each chakra can be particularly effective.

3. Journal Your Experiences

- Keep a journal to record your experiences and any insights gained during chakra meditation. Noting changes in your physical, emotional, and spiritual well-being can help you track your progress.

4. Seek Guidance

- If you're new to chakra meditation, consider seeking guidance from a qualified teacher or using guided meditation resources. Proper guidance can ensure you're practicing effectively and safely.

Conclusion

Chakra meditation is a powerful technique for balancing and aligning the body's energy centers, promoting overall physical, emotional, and spiritual well-being. By understanding the chakras and incorporating practices such as guided visualization, chanting, breathing techniques, affirmations, and crystal healing, you can enhance your meditation practice and experience the profound benefits of chakra balancing. Regular chakra meditation can lead to greater energy balance, improved health, emotional stability, and deeper spiritual growth, enriching your overall meditation journey.

Zen and Vipassana Meditation

Zen and Vipassana are two of the most well-known and respected forms of meditation, each with deep roots in ancient spiritual traditions. Both practices offer unique approaches and benefits, focusing on mindfulness, insight, and the cultivation of a deep sense of peace and clarity. This section explores the principles, techniques, and benefits of Zen and Vipassana meditation, providing guidance on how to incorporate these advanced practices into your meditation routine.

Zen Meditation (Zazen)

1. Overview of Zen Meditation

- Zen meditation, or Zazen, is a cornerstone of Zen Buddhism. It emphasizes sitting meditation and mindfulness to develop deep awareness and insight. Zen meditation focuses on observing the present moment without attachment or judgment.

2. Principles of Zen Meditation

- Mindfulness and Presence: Zen meditation emphasizes being fully present and aware of each moment.

- Non-Attachment: Practitioners are encouraged to observe thoughts and sensations without attachment or identification.

- Simplicity and Discipline: The practice is simple but requires discipline and consistency.

3. Techniques of Zen Meditation

- Posture: Sit on a cushion (zafu) or chair with a straight spine. The traditional posture involves sitting cross-legged in the lotus or half-lotus position, with hands resting in the lap in a cosmic mudra (left hand on top of the right, thumbs lightly touching).

- Breathing: Focus on natural breathing. Pay attention to the sensation of breath entering and leaving the nostrils or the rise and fall of the abdomen.

- Gaze: Keep your eyes open, gazing softly at a point on the floor a few feet in front of you. This helps maintain alertness and prevent drowsiness.

- Thought Observation: Allow thoughts to arise and pass without attachment. When thoughts arise, gently return your focus to your breath or posture.

4. Benefits of Zen Meditation

- Enhanced Mindfulness: Regular practice increases mindfulness and awareness of the present moment.

- Improved Concentration: Zen meditation enhances focus and mental clarity.

- Emotional Regulation: The practice fosters emotional stability and reduces reactivity.

- Spiritual Insight: Zen meditation can lead to profound spiritual insights and a deeper understanding of the nature of existence.

Vipassana Meditation

1. Overview of Vipassana Meditation

- Vipassana, meaning "insight" or "clear seeing," is one of the oldest forms of meditation, originating from the teachings of the Buddha. Vipassana meditation aims to cultivate insight into the true nature of reality through mindfulness and observation.

2. Principles of Vipassana Meditation

- Mindfulness: Central to Vipassana is the cultivation of continuous, non-judgmental mindfulness of thoughts, feelings, and sensations.

- Impermanence: Practitioners observe the impermanent nature of all experiences, fostering a deep understanding of change and non-attachment.

- Suffering and Non-Self: Vipassana aims to understand the nature of suffering and the concept of non-self (Anatta).

3. Techniques of Vipassana Meditation

- Posture: Sit comfortably with a straight spine, either on a cushion or chair. Hands can rest in the lap or on the knees.

- Breath Awareness: Begin with focusing on the breath, observing the natural inhalation and exhalation. Pay attention to the sensation of the breath at the nostrils or the rise and fall of the abdomen.

- Body Scan: Systematically scan the body, observing sensations without reaction. Notice areas of tension, pain, or comfort, and observe them with equanimity.

- Mindfulness of Thoughts and Emotions: Expand awareness to include thoughts and emotions. Observe them as they arise and pass away, noting their impermanent nature.

4. Benefits of Vipassana Meditation

- Deep Insight: Vipassana meditation cultivates profound insight into the nature of reality and the workings of the mind.

- Emotional Healing: The practice helps to release deep-seated emotional patterns and promotes healing.

- Enhanced Awareness: Regular practice increases overall mindfulness and self-awareness.

- Reduced Suffering: By understanding the nature of suffering, practitioners can reduce mental and emotional suffering and develop greater peace and contentment.

Incorporating Zen and Vipassana Meditation into Your Practice

1. Establish a Routine

- Consistency: Set aside a regular time each day for meditation. Consistency is key to developing and deepening your practice.

- Environment: Create a quiet, dedicated space for meditation. Ensure it is free from distractions and conducive to relaxation and focus.

2. Start with Short Sessions

- Begin with shorter sessions (10-15 minutes) and gradually increase the duration as you become more comfortable. Both Zen and Vipassana meditation require patience and persistence.

3. Combine Techniques

- Integrate elements of both Zen and Vipassana meditation into your practice. For example, you can start with a body scan (Vipassana) and then shift to breath awareness and thought observation (Zen).

4. Seek Guidance

- Consider attending meditation retreats or workshops to deepen your understanding and practice. Guided instruction from experienced teachers can provide valuable insights and support.

5. Journal Your Experiences

- Keep a meditation journal to record your experiences, insights, and challenges. Reflecting on your practice can help you track progress and identify areas for growth.

Conclusion

Zen and Vipassana meditation offer profound and transformative practices for developing mindfulness, insight, and spiritual awareness. By understanding the principles and techniques of each tradition, you can incorporate these advanced practices into your meditation routine. Regular practice of Zen and Vipassana meditation can lead to enhanced mental clarity, emotional stability, and a deeper understanding of the nature of reality, enriching your overall meditation journey and contributing to a more mindful and fulfilling life.

Integrating Meditation with Other Practices

Integrating meditation with other practices can enhance its benefits and provide a more holistic approach to well-being. Combining meditation with physical, mental, and spiritual activities can deepen your practice and create a balanced lifestyle. This section explores various ways to integrate meditation with other practices, including yoga, Tai Chi, journaling, creative arts, and mindfulness in daily activities.

Yoga and Meditation

1. Synergy of Yoga and Meditation
- Yoga and meditation complement each other beautifully. While yoga prepares the body and mind for meditation through physical postures and breath control, meditation enhances the mindfulness and inner focus developed during yoga practice.

2. Techniques for Integration
- Start with Yoga: Begin your session with yoga to release physical tension and calm the mind. This prepares you for a deeper meditation experience.
- Meditative Asanas: Incorporate meditative postures like Savasana (Corpse Pose) and Padmasana (Lotus Pose) into your yoga routine to combine physical relaxation with mindfulness.
- Mindful Movement: Practice mindfulness during yoga by focusing on the sensations of each movement and breath, integrating meditation into your physical practice.

3. Benefits
- Enhanced physical flexibility and strength
- Improved mental clarity and focus
- Greater relaxation and stress reduction

Tai Chi and Meditation

1. Principles of Tai Chi
- Tai Chi is a Chinese martial art that involves slow, deliberate movements, deep breathing, and a meditative focus. It emphasizes balance, flow, and the cultivation of life energy (Qi).

2. Techniques for Integration
- Mindful Movements: Practice Tai Chi movements with full awareness of your body, breath, and energy flow, integrating meditation into the physical practice.

- Standing Meditation: Incorporate standing meditation (Zhan Zhuang) into your Tai Chi practice to develop stillness, balance, and inner strength.

- Breath Awareness: Focus on deep, diaphragmatic breathing during Tai Chi to enhance the meditative aspect of the practice.

3. Benefits
- Improved balance and coordination
- Enhanced energy flow and vitality
- Greater mental calm and focus

Journaling and Meditation

1. Reflective Practice

- Journaling is a powerful tool for self-reflection and personal growth. Combining journaling with meditation can deepen your insights and help you process your experiences more effectively.

2. Techniques for Integration

- Pre-Meditation Journaling: Write down your thoughts, feelings, and intentions before meditation to clear your mind and set a focus for your practice.

- Post-Meditation Journaling: Reflect on your meditation experience after your session. Note any insights, emotions, or physical sensations that arose.

- Gratitude Journaling: Incorporate a gratitude practice into your journaling routine to cultivate a positive mindset and enhance your meditation.

3. Benefits

- Increased self-awareness and clarity
- Enhanced emotional processing and healing
- Greater insight and personal growth

Creative Arts and Meditation

1. Art as Meditation

- Creative arts such as drawing, painting, music, and dance can be meditative practices. They engage the mind in a focused, present-moment activity that promotes mindfulness and self-expression.

2. Techniques for Integration

- Mindful Drawing or Painting: Create art with a meditative focus, paying attention to the sensations, colors, and emotions involved in the process.

- Music Meditation: Listen to or create music as a form of meditation. Focus on the sounds, rhythms, and emotions evoked by the music.

- Dance Meditation: Practice mindful movement through dance. Allow your body to move freely and expressively, focusing on the sensations and emotions that arise.

3. Benefits

- Enhanced creativity and self-expression
- Increased mindfulness and present-moment awareness
- Emotional release and relaxation

Mindfulness in Daily Activities

1. Everyday Mindfulness

- Integrating mindfulness into daily activities can transform routine tasks into opportunities for meditation. This practice helps cultivate a continuous state of mindfulness and presence.

2. Techniques for Integration

- Mindful Eating: Pay full attention to the taste, texture, and aroma of your food. Eat slowly and savor each bite, noticing the sensations and emotions associated with eating.

- Mindful Walking: Practice walking meditation by focusing on the sensations of each step, the movement of your body, and your surroundings. Walk slowly and deliberately, bringing your attention to the present moment.

- Mindful Breathing: Incorporate mindful breathing into various activities, such as waiting in line, working, or driving. Focus on your breath to anchor yourself in the present moment.

3. Benefits
- Enhanced awareness and presence
- Reduced stress and improved emotional regulation
- Greater appreciation for daily experiences

Combining Practices for a Holistic Approach

1. Create a Balanced Routine
- Develop a daily or weekly routine that incorporates a variety of practices, such as meditation, yoga, Tai Chi, journaling, and creative arts. This holistic approach can address multiple aspects of your well-being.

2. Listen to Your Body and Mind
- Pay attention to your physical, emotional, and mental needs. Adjust your routine as necessary to ensure it remains supportive and beneficial.

3. Seek Guidance and Support
- Join classes, workshops, or groups to learn new techniques and gain support from others. Guidance from experienced teachers can enhance your practice and provide valuable insights.

Conclusion

Integrating meditation with other practices can create a comprehensive approach to well-being, addressing physical, mental, emotional, and spiritual aspects of your life. By combining meditation with activities such as yoga, Tai Chi, journaling, creative arts, and mindfulness in daily activities, you can deepen your practice and enhance its benefits. This holistic approach fosters greater balance, self-awareness, and overall well-being, enriching your meditation journey and contributing to a more fulfilling and mindful life.

8

Creating a Personal Meditation Routine

Designing Your Schedule

Creating a personal meditation routine tailored to your lifestyle and goals is essential for maintaining consistency and reaping the benefits of regular practice. Designing a schedule that fits seamlessly into your daily life requires thoughtful consideration of your individual needs, preferences, and commitments. This section provides practical advice on how to design a meditation schedule that works for you.

Assessing Your Needs and Goals

1. Identify Your Goals

- Determine what you hope to achieve through meditation. Are you looking to reduce stress, improve focus, enhance emotional well-being, or deepen your spiritual practice? Clearly defining your goals will help shape your meditation routine.

2. Evaluate Your Schedule

- Take an honest look at your daily schedule and identify times when you can realistically fit in meditation. Consider your work, family responsibilities, and other commitments.

3. Consider Your Energy Levels

- Pay attention to your natural energy levels throughout the day. Some people find that meditating in the morning helps set a positive tone for the day, while others prefer evening meditation to unwind and relax before bed.

Choosing the Right Time

1. Morning Meditation

- Benefits: Morning meditation can help you start the day with clarity, focus, and calm. It sets a positive tone and can enhance productivity and mindfulness throughout the day.

- Tips: Set your alarm a bit earlier to create a quiet space for meditation. Start with shorter sessions and gradually increase the duration as you become more comfortable with the routine.

2. Midday Meditation

- Benefits: Meditating during the day can provide a mental reset, reduce stress, and increase energy and focus for the afternoon.

- Tips: Find a quiet space during your lunch break or any free time you have. Even a short 5-10 minute session can be beneficial.

3. Evening Meditation

- Benefits: Evening meditation can help you unwind, release the stress of the day, and promote better sleep. It can also be a time for reflection and gratitude.

- Tips: Choose a consistent time each evening to meditate. Consider integrating meditation into your bedtime routine to signal to your body that it's time to relax and prepare for sleep.

Determining the Frequency and Duration

1. Start Small

- Begin with short sessions, such as 5-10 minutes, especially if you are new to meditation. This makes it easier to commit to the practice and prevents feelings of overwhelm.

2. Gradual Increase

- As you become more comfortable with meditation, gradually increase the duration of your sessions. Aim for 20-30 minutes per session for deeper benefits.

3. Daily Practice

- Consistency is key. Aim to meditate daily, even if some days you can only manage a few minutes. Regular practice helps build the habit and ensures long-term benefits.

Incorporating Different Meditation Techniques

1. Variety in Practice

- Incorporate different meditation techniques into your routine to keep it engaging and address various aspects of well-being. Mix mindfulness meditation, loving-kindness meditation, body scan, and breath-focused meditation.

2. Weekly Themes

- Consider setting weekly themes for your meditation practice. For example, focus on stress relief one week, emotional healing the next, and enhancing focus the following week.

Creating a Supportive Environment

1. Designate a Meditation Space

- Choose a quiet, comfortable space in your home dedicated to meditation. Having a specific spot helps create a conducive environment and reinforces the habit.

2. Minimize Distractions

- Ensure your meditation space is free from distractions. Turn off electronic devices, close the door, and inform family members of your meditation time to avoid interruptions.

3. Personalize Your Space

- Make your meditation space inviting by adding cushions, blankets, candles, or calming artwork. Personal touches can enhance your practice and make it more enjoyable.

Tracking Your Progress

1. Meditation Journal

- Keep a meditation journal to record your sessions, noting the duration, techniques used, and any insights or experiences. Reflecting on your practice helps track progress and identify patterns or areas for improvement.

2. Use Meditation Apps

- Many meditation apps offer features to track your progress, such as session logs, streaks, and milestones. Using these tools can provide motivation and a sense of achievement.

Adapting to Changes

1. Flexibility

- Be flexible with your routine. Life circumstances may change, and it's important to adapt your meditation schedule accordingly. The key is to maintain consistency, even if the timing or duration of your sessions varies.

2. Self-Compassion

- Approach your meditation practice with self-compassion. It's normal to miss a session occasionally or have days when meditation feels challenging. Be kind to yourself and gently return to your practice without judgment.

Conclusion

Designing a personal meditation schedule involves assessing your needs and goals, choosing the right time for practice, determining the frequency and duration, incorporating different techniques, creating a supportive environment, tracking your progress, and being flexible with changes. By thoughtfully considering these factors, you can create a meditation routine that fits seamlessly into your daily life, enhances your well-being, and helps you achieve your meditation goals. Regular, consistent practice is the foundation for experiencing the profound benefits of meditation and fostering a lifelong habit of mindfulness and inner peace.

Tracking Your Progress

Tracking your progress in meditation is crucial for maintaining motivation, understanding your growth, and refining your practice. By systematically observing and recording your meditation experiences, you can gain insights into your progress, identify areas for improvement, and celebrate milestones. This section explores various methods and tools for tracking your meditation progress effectively.

The Importance of Tracking Your Progress

1. Motivation and Accountability

- Tracking your progress helps maintain motivation by providing tangible evidence of your commitment and improvement. It also holds you accountable to your practice, making it more likely that you will stick with it.

2. Insight and Reflection

- Keeping records of your meditation experiences allows for deeper reflection and insight. It helps you identify patterns, recognize changes in your mental and emotional states, and understand what techniques work best for you.

3. Celebrating Milestones

- Recognizing and celebrating milestones can boost your confidence and reinforce the positive impact of meditation. Tracking your progress makes it easier to see how far you've come and appreciate your achievements.

Methods for Tracking Your Meditation Progress

1. Meditation Journal

2. Regular Entries

- Keep a dedicated meditation journal where you record details about each session. Include the date, time, duration, technique used, and any notable experiences or insights. Regular entries help you track your consistency and progress over time.

3. Reflection Questions

- Include reflection questions in your journal to deepen your self-awareness. Questions can include:
  - How did I feel before and after the session?
  - What thoughts or emotions arose during meditation?
  - Were there any physical sensations or discomforts?
  - What insights or realizations did I have?
  - How can I apply these insights to my daily life?

4. Gratitude Practice

- Incorporate a gratitude practice into your journaling routine. Reflect on and write down things you are grateful for, both in your meditation practice and in your daily life. This practice can enhance your overall well-being and positive outlook.

Using Meditation Apps

1. Tracking Features

- Many meditation apps offer built-in tracking features that log your sessions, including duration, frequency, and techniques used. Apps like Headspace, Calm, and Insight Timer provide detailed statistics and visual representations of your progress.

2. Reminders and Streaks

- Utilize reminders and streak features to maintain consistency. Apps can send notifications to remind you to meditate and track streaks to motivate you to keep up with your practice.

3. Guided Meditations

- Follow guided meditations available on apps and track how different sessions impact your mental and emotional state. Guided sessions can provide variety and structure to your practice.

Creating Visual Charts and Graphs

1. Progress Charts

- Create visual charts to track your meditation sessions. Use a calendar or chart to mark each day you meditate. Seeing your progress visually can be motivating and provide a clear picture of your consistency.

2. Graphing Duration and Frequency

- Use graphs to track the duration and frequency of your meditation sessions over time. Plotting these metrics can help you identify patterns and trends in your practice.

3. Mood and Energy Levels

- Track your mood and energy levels before and after each session. Create a simple rating scale (e.g., 1-10) to quantify how you feel. Over time, you can analyze how meditation affects your overall well-being.

Reflecting on Milestones and Achievements

1. Setting Goals

- Set specific, achievable goals for your meditation practice, such as meditating for a certain number of minutes each day, completing a series of guided sessions, or reaching a particular streak. Write down these goals and track your progress towards them.

2. Celebrating Achievements

- Celebrate your milestones, such as completing a month of daily meditation, reaching a new duration record, or experiencing a significant insight. Acknowledge your efforts and reward yourself for your dedication.

3. Review and Adjust

- Periodically review your meditation journal, app logs, and visual charts. Reflect on your progress and adjust your practice as needed. Identify what's working well and what could be improved, and set new goals to keep your practice evolving.

Seeking Feedback and Support

1. Meditation Groups and Communities
- Join meditation groups or online communities where you can share your experiences and progress. Engaging with others can provide support, encouragement, and new perspectives on your practice.

2. Mentorship and Guidance
- Seek feedback and guidance from experienced meditators or teachers. They can offer valuable insights, help you refine your technique, and provide support as you navigate challenges.

3. Accountability Partners
- Partner with a friend or family member who also meditates. Share your goals and progress with each other, and provide mutual support and accountability.

Conclusion

Tracking your progress is a vital component of creating and maintaining a personal meditation routine. By using methods such as journaling, meditation apps, visual charts, and seeking feedback, you can gain valuable insights, stay motivated, and celebrate your achievements. Regularly reflecting on your progress and adjusting your practice ensures that you continue to grow and benefit from meditation. With dedication and a structured approach to tracking, you can deepen your meditation practice and enhance your overall well-being.

Adjusting Your Practice

As you progress in your meditation journey, you may find that your needs and preferences evolve. Adjusting your practice to accommodate these changes is essential for maintaining a sustainable and effective meditation routine. This section provides guidance on how to adapt your meditation practice to ensure it continues to meet your goals, remains engaging, and supports your overall well-being.

Recognizing the Need for Adjustment

1. Identifying Stagnation

- If you feel that your meditation practice has become routine or stagnant, it may be time to make adjustments. Signs of stagnation include a lack of engagement, decreased motivation, or feeling that your practice is no longer yielding the desired benefits.

2. Addressing Challenges

- Challenges such as increased stress, changes in your schedule, or shifts in your emotional state may require adjustments to your practice. Recognize these challenges as opportunities to refine and enhance your meditation routine.

3. Listening to Your Intuition

- Trust your intuition and inner guidance. If you feel drawn to explore new techniques or modify your practice, honor that impulse. Meditation is a personal journey, and your practice should reflect your unique needs and experiences.

Incorporating New Techniques

1. Exploring Different Styles

- Experiment with different meditation styles to keep your practice fresh and engaging. Try mindfulness meditation, loving-kindness meditation, body scan, transcendental meditation, or guided visualization. Each style offers unique benefits and can enhance your overall practice.

2. Integrating Advanced Practices

- As you become more experienced, consider incorporating advanced practices such as Zen meditation, Vipassana meditation, or chakra meditation. These techniques can deepen your practice and provide new insights and experiences.

3. Combining Practices

- Integrate meditation with other practices such as yoga, Tai Chi, journaling, or creative arts. Combining these activities can create a holistic routine that supports physical, mental, and emotional well-being.

Adapting to Changes in Schedule

1. Flexible Timing

- Be flexible with the timing of your meditation sessions. If your schedule changes, adjust your practice accordingly. The key is to maintain consistency, even if the timing or duration varies.

2. Shorter Sessions

- If you find it challenging to fit longer sessions into your day, opt for shorter, more frequent sessions. Even a few minutes of meditation can be beneficial and help maintain your practice.

3. Integrating Meditation into Daily Activities

- Practice mindfulness during daily activities such as walking, eating, or working. Integrating meditation into these moments can help you stay connected to your practice and promote mindfulness throughout the day.

Responding to Emotional and Physical Changes

1. Tailoring Techniques to Your State

- Adjust your meditation techniques based on your current emotional and physical state. For example, if you are feeling anxious, focus on calming breathwork or guided relaxation. If you are feeling low energy, try a more active meditation such as walking meditation.

2. Self-Compassion and Patience

- Approach changes in your practice with self-compassion and patience. It's normal to experience fluctuations in motivation and engagement. Be kind to yourself and allow for adjustments without judgment.

3. Regular Check-Ins

- Periodically check in with yourself to assess how your practice is aligning with your goals and needs. Reflect on what's working well and what might need adjustment. These regular check-ins can help you stay attuned to your evolving practice.

Seeking Guidance and Support

1. Meditation Teachers and Mentors

- Seek guidance from experienced meditation teachers or mentors. They can provide valuable insights, suggest new techniques, and offer support as you navigate changes in your practice.

2. Community and Group Practice

- Join a meditation group or community to share experiences and gain support from others. Group practice can introduce new perspectives and techniques that enrich your individual practice.

3. Continuing Education

- Participate in workshops, retreats, or courses to deepen your understanding of meditation and explore advanced practices. Continued learning can inspire and invigorate your practice.

Setting New Goals

1. Revisiting Your Intentions

- Regularly revisit your intentions and goals for meditation. As your life evolves, your goals may change. Adjust your practice to align with your current aspirations and needs.

2. Setting Short-Term and Long-Term Goals

- Establish both short-term and long-term goals for your practice. Short-term goals provide immediate focus and motivation, while long-term goals guide your overall journey.

3. Tracking Progress

- Continue to track your progress and reflect on your achievements. Celebrate milestones and use them as motivation to keep moving forward. Regularly setting and reassessing goals helps maintain direction and purpose in your practice.

Conclusion

Adjusting your meditation practice is a natural and necessary part of maintaining a sustainable and effective routine. By recognizing the need for change, incorporating new techniques, adapting to schedule shifts, responding to emotional and physical changes, seeking guidance, and setting new goals, you can ensure that your practice remains dynamic and supportive of your overall well-being. Embrace the flexibility and personal nature of meditation, allowing your practice to evolve and grow with you. This adaptability will help you continue to experience the profound benefits of meditation and maintain a lifelong habit of mindfulness and inner peace.

9

Meditation in Daily Life

Mindfulness in Everyday Activities

Integrating mindfulness into everyday activities is a powerful way to bring the benefits of meditation into your daily life. Mindfulness involves paying full attention to the present moment, with an attitude of openness and non-judgment. Practicing mindfulness in daily tasks can enhance your overall well-being, reduce stress, and increase your sense of presence and fulfillment. This section explores practical strategies for incorporating mindfulness into various everyday activities.

Understanding Mindfulness

1. Definition of Mindfulness

   - Mindfulness is the practice of being fully present and engaged in the current moment, observing your thoughts, feelings, and sensations without judgment. It involves an attitude of curiosity and acceptance, allowing you to experience life more deeply and authentically.

2. Benefits of Mindfulness in Daily Life

- Reduced Stress: Mindfulness helps to break the cycle of stress by promoting relaxation and emotional regulation.

- Improved Focus and Concentration: Practicing mindfulness enhances your ability to concentrate and stay focused on tasks.

- Enhanced Emotional Well-Being: Mindfulness fosters greater self-awareness and emotional intelligence, leading to improved relationships and overall happiness.

Mindful Eating

1. Slow Down

- Take your time when eating, savoring each bite. Chew slowly and focus on the texture, taste, and aroma of your food. Eating mindfully helps you appreciate your meal and promotes better digestion.

2. Engage Your Senses

- Use all your senses to fully experience your food. Notice the colors, shapes, and smells of your meal. Pay attention to the sounds of chewing and the sensations in your mouth and body as you eat.

3. Gratitude and Intention

- Before eating, take a moment to express gratitude for your food. Reflect on where it came from and the effort that went into its preparation. Setting an intention for your meal can enhance your mindfulness practice.

Mindful Walking

1. Focus on Your Steps

- Pay attention to the sensation of your feet touching the ground with each step. Notice the rhythm of your walk and the movement of your legs and body. Walking mindfully can turn an everyday activity into a meditative practice.

2. Observe Your Surroundings

- Be fully present to your environment as you walk. Notice the sights, sounds, and smells around you. Engage with the natural world by observing the sky, trees, and wildlife.

3. Breath Awareness

- Coordinate your breath with your steps. For example, take a deep breath in for three steps and exhale for the next three steps. This synchronization helps anchor your mind and enhances your mindfulness.

Mindful Working

1. Single-Tasking

- Focus on one task at a time, giving it your full attention. Avoid multitasking, which can divide your attention and reduce your effectiveness. Mindful working enhances productivity and job satisfaction.

2. Take Breaks

- Incorporate short mindfulness breaks throughout your workday. Use these breaks to stretch, take a few deep breaths, or practice a brief meditation. These moments of mindfulness can recharge your energy and improve your focus.

3. Mindful Listening

- Practice active listening in your interactions with colleagues. Give your full attention to the speaker, avoid interrupting, and respond thoughtfully. Mindful listening fosters better communication and relationships.

Mindful Cleaning

1. Focus on the Task

- Pay attention to the physical sensations involved in cleaning, such as the feel of the cloth, the smell of the cleaning products, and the movements of your body. Mindful cleaning transforms a routine chore into a meditative activity.

2. Set an Intention

- Approach cleaning with a positive mindset and set an intention for the task. For example, you might focus on creating a clean and peaceful environment or use the time to clear your mind.

3. Be Present

- Stay present and engaged in the cleaning process. Avoid letting your mind wander to other tasks or worries. This practice helps you cultivate mindfulness and appreciate the sense of accomplishment that comes with a clean space.

Mindful Communication

1. Be Present

- Give your full attention to the person you are communicating with. Avoid distractions such as checking your phone or thinking about your response while the other person is speaking.

2. Practice Empathy

- Listen with empathy and try to understand the other person's perspective. This practice fosters deeper connections and more meaningful interactions.

3. Respond Thoughtfully

- Take a moment to pause and reflect before responding. This pause allows you to choose your words mindfully and communicate more effectively and compassionately.

Mindful Driving

1. Stay Focused

- Pay full attention to the act of driving. Notice the feel of the steering wheel, the sounds of the car, and the movement of the vehicle. Avoid distractions such as checking your phone or eating while driving.

2. Practice Patience

- Use driving as an opportunity to practice patience and mindfulness. If you encounter traffic or delays, take a few deep breaths and focus on staying calm and present.

3. Observe Your Surroundings

- Be aware of your surroundings and stay present to the road and other drivers. Mindful driving enhances safety and reduces stress.

Incorporating Mindfulness into Daily Routines

1. Morning Routine

- Start your day with mindfulness. Incorporate a brief meditation, mindful stretching, or deep breathing into your morning routine. Setting a mindful tone for the day can influence your overall mindset and well-being.

2. Evening Routine

- End your day with mindfulness. Reflect on the day's experiences, practice gratitude, and engage in calming activities such as reading or meditating. An evening mindfulness practice can promote better sleep and relaxation.

3. Mindful Transitions

- Use transitions between activities as opportunities for mindfulness. Take a few moments to breathe and center yourself before moving on to the next task. These mindful pauses can help you stay present and focused throughout the day.

Conclusion

Integrating mindfulness into everyday activities is a powerful way to extend the benefits of meditation into all aspects of your life. By practicing mindfulness in activities such as eating, walking, working, cleaning, communicating, and driving, you can enhance your overall well-being, reduce stress, and cultivate a deeper sense of presence and fulfillment. Making mindfulness a part of your daily routine helps create a more mindful, balanced, and enriched life, allowing you to experience each moment fully and authentically.

Dealing with Stress and Challenges

Life is filled with stressors and challenges that can affect your mental and emotional well-being. Incorporating meditation and mindfulness into your daily routine can help you manage stress more effectively, build resilience, and navigate challenges with greater ease. This section explores strategies for using meditation and mindfulness to deal with stress and challenges, offering practical techniques to help you maintain balance and inner peace.

Understanding Stress and Its Impact

1. Definition of Stress
   - Stress is the body's response to perceived threats or challenges. It triggers the release of hormones such as cortisol and adrenaline, preparing the body for a "fight or flight" response. While some stress is normal and can be motivating, chronic stress can have negative effects on your health and well-being.

2. Effects of Chronic Stress
   - Physical Health: Chronic stress can lead to headaches, muscle tension, digestive issues, and weakened immune function.
   - Mental Health: Prolonged stress can contribute to anxiety, depression, irritability, and difficulty concentrating.

- Emotional Health: Ongoing stress can result in feelings of overwhelm, frustration, and burnout.

Using Meditation to Manage Stress

1. Mindfulness Meditation

- Technique: Sit comfortably, close your eyes, and focus on your breath. Notice each inhalation and exhalation, bringing your attention back to your breath whenever your mind wanders.

- Benefits: Mindfulness meditation helps calm the mind, reduce anxiety, and improve emotional regulation by promoting present-moment awareness and non-judgmental observation of thoughts and feelings.

2. Body Scan Meditation

- Technique: Lie down or sit comfortably. Slowly scan your body from head to toe, paying attention to any sensations, tension, or areas of discomfort. Breathe into each area, allowing tension to release.

- Benefits: Body scan meditation helps to release physical tension, promote relaxation, and increase body awareness, reducing the physical impact of stress.

3. Loving-Kindness Meditation

- Technique: Sit comfortably and close your eyes. Silently repeat phrases such as "May I be happy, may I be healthy, may I be safe, may I live with ease." Gradually extend these wishes to others, including loved ones, acquaintances, and even those with whom you have conflicts.

- Benefits: Loving-kindness meditation fosters compassion and empathy, reduces negative emotions, and promotes positive social connections, helping to counteract the effects of stress.

Practical Techniques for Dealing with Stress

1. Breath Control and Deep Breathing
   - Technique: Practice deep, diaphragmatic breathing. Inhale deeply through your nose, allowing your abdomen to expand, and exhale slowly through your mouth.
   - Benefits: Deep breathing activates the body's relaxation response, reducing stress hormones and promoting a sense of calm.

2. Progressive Muscle Relaxation
   - Technique: Tense and then relax each muscle group in your body, starting from your toes and moving up to your head. Focus on the contrast between tension and relaxation.
   - Benefits: Progressive muscle relaxation helps release physical tension, reduce anxiety, and promote overall relaxation.

3. Visualization and Guided Imagery
   - Technique: Close your eyes and imagine a peaceful, calming scene, such as a beach, forest, or mountain. Engage all your senses to make the visualization vivid and immersive.
   - Benefits: Visualization and guided imagery can reduce stress, promote relaxation, and provide a mental escape from stressful situations.

Mindfulness Practices for Navigating Challenges

1. Mindful Awareness
   - Technique: Practice being fully present and aware during challenging situations. Notice your thoughts, emotions, and physical sensations without judgment. Acknowledge your feelings and allow them to pass

without reacting impulsively.

- Benefits: Mindful awareness helps you respond to challenges with greater clarity and composure, reducing reactive behavior and improving problem-solving skills.

2. Acceptance and Non-Judgment

- Technique: Cultivate an attitude of acceptance and non-judgment towards yourself and the situation. Acknowledge that challenges are a natural part of life and that it's okay to feel stressed or overwhelmed.

- Benefits: Acceptance and non-judgment reduce resistance and negative self-talk, promoting a more balanced and compassionate approach to challenges.

3. Mindful Reflection

- Technique: Reflect on challenging situations with a mindful perspective. Consider what you can learn from the experience and how you can apply this knowledge in the future.

- Benefits: Mindful reflection fosters personal growth, resilience, and a more positive outlook on life's challenges.

Integrating Mindfulness into Daily Activities

1. Mindful Morning Routine

- Start your day with mindfulness practices such as deep breathing, meditation, or setting intentions. This sets a positive tone for the day and helps you approach challenges with a calm and focused mindset.

2. Mindful Breaks

- Take short mindfulness breaks throughout the day. Practice deep breathing, body scans, or simply observe your surroundings. These breaks help reset your mind and reduce accumulated stress.

3. Mindful Evening Routine

- End your day with mindfulness practices such as reflection, gratitude journaling, or gentle yoga. This helps release the day's stress and promotes restful sleep.

Building Resilience Through Meditation

1. Regular Practice

- Consistency is key to building resilience. Make meditation and mindfulness a regular part of your daily routine to cultivate a stable foundation for managing stress and challenges.

2. Adaptability

- Be adaptable in your practice. Adjust your meditation techniques and mindfulness practices to suit your current needs and circumstances. Flexibility ensures that your practice remains effective and supportive.

3. Community and Support

- Engage with meditation groups or communities for support and encouragement. Sharing experiences and learning from others can enhance your practice and provide valuable insights for managing stress.

Conclusion

Dealing with stress and challenges is an inevitable part of life, but incorporating meditation and mindfulness into your daily routine can help you manage these experiences more effectively. By practicing mindfulness in everyday activities, using specific meditation techniques, and building resilience through regular practice, you can reduce stress, enhance emotional well-being, and navigate challenges with greater ease and clarity. Embracing these practices can lead to a more balanced, peaceful, and fulfilling life.

Cultivating a Meditative Lifestyle

Cultivating a meditative lifestyle means integrating the principles and practices of meditation into all aspects of your daily life. This approach extends the benefits of meditation beyond formal practice sessions, fostering a continuous state of mindfulness, presence, and inner peace. This section explores strategies for embedding meditation into your lifestyle, helping you maintain a balanced and mindful approach to everyday living.

Embracing Mindfulness in Daily Routines

1. Morning Rituals

- Mindful Waking: Start your day with a few moments of mindful breathing or a short meditation before getting out of bed. This sets a calm and focused tone for the day.

- Morning Gratitude: Upon waking, take a moment to express gratitude for a new day and set a positive intention.

2. Daily Activities

- Mindful Eating: Practice eating with full attention. Savor each bite, notice the flavors and textures, and eat slowly. This promotes better digestion and a more satisfying eating experience.

- Mindful Walking: Use your daily walks as opportunities for mindfulness. Focus on the sensation of your feet touching the ground, the rhythm of your breath, and the sights and sounds around you.

3. Work and Productivity

- Focused Work: Apply mindfulness to your work by focusing on one task at a time. Avoid multitasking and give your full attention to each activity. Take short breaks to practice mindful breathing or stretching to maintain focus and reduce stress.

- Mindful Communication: Engage in active listening and present-moment awareness during conversations with colleagues and clients. This fosters better relationships and more effective communication.

Creating a Meditative Environment

1. Home Space

- Designated Meditation Area: Set aside a specific area in your home for meditation. Keep this space clean, uncluttered, and dedicated to your practice. Personalize it with items that promote relaxation, such as cushions, candles, or plants.

- Mindful Decor: Decorate your living space with calming colors, natural elements, and minimalistic designs to create a peaceful and mindful atmosphere.

2. Work Space

- Clutter-Free Desk: Keep your workspace organized and free of clutter to enhance focus and productivity. Incorporate calming elements such as a small plant, a calming photo, or a stress-relief object.

- Break Spaces: Create a quiet corner in your workplace where you can take mindful breaks. Use this space for short meditation sessions or deep breathing exercises to reset and recharge.

Mindful Relationships

1. Quality Time

- Mindful Presence: Be fully present with your loved ones. Listen actively, engage in meaningful conversations, and show appreciation and gratitude. Avoid distractions such as checking your phone during interactions.

- Shared Activities: Engage in activities that promote connection and mindfulness, such as cooking together, going for walks, or practicing meditation as a family.

2. Compassion and Empathy

- Loving-Kindness Practice: Regularly practice loving-kindness meditation to cultivate compassion and empathy towards yourself and others. This can enhance your relationships and promote a sense of interconnectedness.

- Conflict Resolution: Approach conflicts with a mindful and non-reactive attitude. Practice active listening, express your feelings calmly, and seek mutually beneficial solutions.

Balancing Digital Life

1. Digital Detox

- Scheduled Breaks: Allocate specific times during the day to disconnect from digital devices. Use these breaks for mindful activities such as reading, walking, or meditating.

- Mindful Use: Set intentions for your digital use. Be mindful of the time spent on devices and choose content that supports your well-being and growth.

2. Online Mindfulness

- Mindful Browsing: Apply mindfulness to your online activities. Be aware of how you engage with digital content and notice any emotional responses it triggers. Take breaks if you feel overwhelmed or distracted.

- Virtual Meditation: Participate in online meditation sessions or mindfulness courses. These can provide structure, community, and support for your practice.

Integrating Mindfulness into Leisure Activities

1. Hobbies and Interests

- Mindful Engagement: Engage in hobbies and activities with full attention and presence. Whether it's gardening, painting, playing music, or cooking, immerse yourself in the experience and enjoy the process.

- Creative Expression: Use creative activities as a form of meditation. Focus on the sensations, emotions, and thoughts that arise during the creative process.

2. Nature Connection

- Outdoor Meditation: Practice meditation in natural settings such as parks, forests, or near water. Nature's tranquility can enhance your practice and deepen your connection to the present moment.

- Eco-Mindfulness: Cultivate a mindful relationship with the environment. Practice eco-friendly habits, appreciate nature's beauty, and engage in activities that promote environmental sustainability.

Practicing Self-Care and Compassion

1. Regular Self-Care

- Mindful Self-Care: Incorporate mindfulness into your self-care routine. Pay attention to your body's needs, engage in activities that nourish your mind and spirit, and prioritize rest and relaxation.

- Body Awareness: Practice mindful body awareness through activities such as yoga, Tai Chi, or gentle stretching. These practices promote physical well-being and deepen your connection to your body.

2. Self-Compassion

- Kindness to Yourself: Treat yourself with the same compassion and understanding that you would offer to a friend. Acknowledge your efforts, forgive your mistakes, and celebrate your successes.

- Compassionate Reflection: Reflect on your experiences with a compassionate perspective. Recognize your growth and learning, and be gentle with yourself during challenging times.

Conclusion

Cultivating a meditative lifestyle involves integrating mindfulness and meditation into all aspects of your daily life. By embracing mindfulness in your routines, creating a meditative environment, fostering mindful relationships, balancing digital life, engaging in mindful leisure activities, and practicing self-care and compassion, you can maintain a state of continuous presence and inner peace. This holistic approach not only enhances the benefits of your meditation practice but also promotes a more balanced, fulfilling, and enriched life. By living mindfully, you can experience greater well-being, resilience, and joy in every moment.

10

Resources and Further Reading

Recommended Books and Authors

Exploring additional resources can deepen your understanding of meditation and mindfulness, offering new insights and techniques to enhance your practice. This section provides a list of recommended books and authors that are highly regarded in the field of meditation, mindfulness, and spiritual growth. These works can serve as valuable guides on your journey towards greater mindfulness and inner peace.

Foundational Texts on Meditation and Mindfulness

1. "The Miracle of Mindfulness" by Thich Nhat Hanh
 - Overview: This classic book by Vietnamese Zen master Thich Nhat Hanh introduces mindfulness as a way of living. It offers practical exercises and gentle reminders to bring mindfulness into daily activities.

- Why Read It: Thich Nhat Hanh's simple yet profound teachings are accessible to beginners and provide a solid foundation for integrating mindfulness into everyday life.

2. "Wherever You Go, There You Are" by Jon Kabat-Zinn

- Overview: Jon Kabat-Zinn, the founder of Mindfulness-Based Stress Reduction (MBSR), presents mindfulness as a way to fully engage with life. The book includes practical guidance and personal anecdotes.

- Why Read It: This book is an excellent introduction to mindfulness and meditation, offering insights and techniques that are easy to incorporate into daily life.

3. "The Power of Now" by Eckhart Tolle

- Overview: Eckhart Tolle explores the concept of living in the present moment and how it can transform your life. The book emphasizes the importance of transcending ego-based thinking.

- Why Read It: Tolle's teachings offer a deep understanding of mindfulness and presence, making it a transformative read for those seeking spiritual growth.

In-Depth Exploration of Meditation Practices

1. "The Art of Happiness" by the Dalai Lama and Howard Cutler

- Overview: This book combines the Dalai Lama's wisdom with insights from Western psychology. It explores how mindfulness and meditation can lead to lasting happiness.

- Why Read It: The practical advice and philosophical insights make this book a valuable resource for understanding the connection between meditation and happiness.

2. "Real Happiness: The Power of Meditation" by Sharon Salzberg

- Overview: Sharon Salzberg, a leading meditation teacher, offers a 28-day program to help readers start and maintain a meditation practice. The book includes guided meditations and practical tips.

- Why Read It: This book is perfect for beginners who want a structured approach to developing a meditation practice.

3. "The Book of Joy" by Dalai Lama, Desmond Tutu, and Douglas Abrams

- Overview: This book captures a week-long conversation between the Dalai Lama and Archbishop Desmond Tutu about finding joy in the face of life's challenges. It includes practical exercises and reflections.

- Why Read It: The wisdom and humor of these two spiritual leaders provide deep insights into cultivating joy and mindfulness.

Exploring the Science of Meditation

1. "The Relaxation Response" by Herbert Benson

- Overview: Dr. Herbert Benson introduces the relaxation response, a scientifically validated method for reducing stress through meditation. The book explains the physiological benefits of meditation.

- Why Read It: This book provides a scientific perspective on meditation, making it a great read for those interested in the health benefits of mindfulness practices.

2. "Altered Traits: Science Reveals How Meditation Changes Your Mind, Brain, and Body" by Daniel Goleman and Richard J. Davidson

- Overview: This book explores the long-term effects of meditation on the brain and body, drawing on cutting-edge research and decades of study.

- Why Read It: The authors present compelling evidence on how meditation can lead to lasting changes in mental and physical health.

3. "The Mindful Brain: Reflection and Attunement in the Cultivation of Well-Being" by Daniel J. Siegel

- Overview: Dr. Daniel Siegel explores the relationship between mindfulness and the brain. The book delves into how mindfulness practices can enhance emotional regulation and overall well-being.

- Why Read It: Siegel's interdisciplinary approach combines neuroscience, psychology, and mindfulness, offering a comprehensive understanding of how meditation affects the brain.

Guides to Advanced Meditation Practices

1. "The Heart of the Buddha's Teaching" by Thich Nhat Hanh

- Overview: Thich Nhat Hanh provides an in-depth exploration of Buddhist teachings and practices, including meditation. The book offers practical advice for integrating these teachings into daily life.

- Why Read It: This book is a valuable resource for those looking to deepen their understanding of Buddhist meditation and philosophy.

2. "Mindfulness in Plain English" by Bhante Henepola Gunaratana

- Overview: Bhante Gunaratana offers a clear and comprehensive guide to mindfulness and Vipassana meditation. The book includes detailed instructions and insights into the practice.

- Why Read It: The straightforward and practical approach makes this book an essential read for anyone serious about developing their meditation practice.

3. "The Places That Scare You: A Guide to Fearlessness in Difficult Times" by Pema Chödrön

- Overview: Pema Chödrön, a renowned Buddhist nun and teacher, explores how to use meditation and mindfulness to face fear and adversity with courage and compassion.

- Why Read It: Chödrön's teachings are particularly helpful for those looking to use meditation as a tool for personal growth and resilience in challenging times.

Contemporary Voices and Practical Guides

1. "10% Happier" by Dan Harris

- Overview: ABC news anchor Dan Harris shares his personal journey with meditation, offering practical advice for skeptics and beginners. The book includes insights from interviews with leading meditation teachers.

- Why Read It: Harris's relatable and humorous approach makes meditation accessible to those who may be skeptical or new to the practice.

2. "Radical Acceptance: Embracing Your Life With the Heart of a Buddha" by Tara Brach

- Overview: Tara Brach combines mindfulness and compassion to explore how to accept ourselves fully. The book includes practical exercises and guided meditations.

- Why Read It: Brach's compassionate and insightful approach provides valuable tools for self-acceptance and healing.

3. "The Headspace Guide to Meditation and Mindfulness" by Andy Puddicombe

- Overview: Andy Puddicombe, the co-founder of Headspace, offers a guide to mindfulness and meditation, including practical tips and guided exercises.

- Why Read It: The easy-to-follow advice and engaging style make this book a great introduction to mindfulness and meditation for beginners.

Conclusion

Exploring the works of these recommended authors and books can significantly enhance your meditation practice and deepen your understanding of mindfulness. Whether you are a beginner looking for practical guidance or an experienced practitioner seeking advanced techniques, these resources offer valuable insights and tools to support your journey. By incorporating these teachings into your daily life, you can cultivate greater mindfulness, inner peace, and overall well-being.

Online Courses and Communities

In today's digital age, numerous online courses and communities can support and enhance your meditation practice. These resources provide access to guided meditations, instructional videos, forums, and support groups, making it easier to maintain a consistent practice and connect with like-minded individuals. This section explores some of the best online courses and communities for meditation and mindfulness.

Online Meditation Courses

1. Headspace

- Overview: Headspace offers a comprehensive library of guided meditations, mindfulness exercises, and sleep aids. The app is designed for beginners and experienced meditators alike, with structured programs and courses on various topics.
- Features:
- Guided meditations for stress, sleep, focus, and anxiety
- Themed meditation courses (e.g., work, relationships, health)
- Short, everyday mindfulness exercises
- Why Use It: Headspace's user-friendly interface and extensive library make it an excellent resource for those looking to integrate meditation into their daily lives.

2. Calm

- Overview: Calm provides a wide range of meditation and relaxation tools, including guided meditations, breathing exercises, and sleep stories. The app caters to all levels of experience and offers specialized programs.
- Features:
- Daily Calm sessions for morning and evening
- Multi-day meditation programs (e.g., 7 Days of Calm, 21 Days of Calm)
- Nature sounds and sleep stories for relaxation
- Why Use It: Calm's variety of content and soothing interface make it a great option for those seeking to reduce stress and improve sleep through meditation.

3. Insight Timer

- Overview: Insight Timer offers a vast collection of free guided meditations from teachers worldwide. The app includes features for tracking your practice and connecting with a global community of meditators.
  - Features:
  - Over 100,000 free guided meditations
  - Customizable meditation timer
  - Courses on mindfulness, self-compassion, and more
- Why Use It: Insight Timer's extensive library and community features make it an ideal resource for finding diverse meditation styles and connecting with others.

4. 10% Happier

- Overview: Founded by Dan Harris, 10% Happier provides practical meditation courses and expert guidance tailored for skeptics and beginners. The app features content from renowned meditation teachers.
  - Features:
  - Video and audio meditation courses
  - Daily meditation reminders and prompts
  - Personal coaching and feedback
- Why Use It: The approachable, no-nonsense style of 10% Happier makes it particularly suitable for those new to meditation or skeptical about its benefits.

5. Mindful Schools

- Overview: Mindful Schools offers online courses for educators, parents, and individuals interested in integrating mindfulness into their daily lives and work. The courses are designed to provide practical mindfulness skills.

- Features:
- Online courses on mindfulness fundamentals, self-compassion, and resilience
    - Specialized programs for educators and parents
    - Access to a supportive online community
    - Why Use It: Mindful Schools' focus on practical application makes it an excellent resource for those looking to bring mindfulness into their personal and professional lives.

Online Meditation Communities

1. Reddit - r/Meditation
    - Overview: r/Meditation is a popular subreddit where users share their meditation experiences, ask questions, and provide support. The community is open to meditators of all levels.
    - Features:
    - Discussion threads on various meditation techniques
    - Daily meditation challenges and prompts
    - Resources for beginners and advanced practitioners
    - Why Use It: The active and supportive community on r/Meditation makes it a valuable resource for finding advice, sharing experiences, and staying motivated.

2. The Mindfulness Meditation Group on Facebook
    - Overview: This Facebook group is dedicated to mindfulness meditation practice. Members share tips, experiences, and resources related to meditation and mindfulness.
    - Features:
    - Regular posts and discussions on mindfulness topics
    - Live guided meditation sessions

- Access to a global community of mindfulness practitioners
- Why Use It: The Mindfulness Meditation Group provides a supportive environment for connecting with others and deepening your practice through shared experiences.

3. Insight Timer Community Groups

- Overview: Insight Timer offers various community groups within the app, where users can join discussions, participate in challenges, and connect with others interested in similar topics.
- Features:
- Topic-specific groups (e.g., anxiety, sleep, self-love)
- Meditation challenges and group events
- Interaction with meditation teachers and practitioners
- Why Use It: The diverse range of groups on Insight Timer allows you to find a community that aligns with your interests and needs, enhancing your meditation practice.

4. Mindful Living Collective

- Overview: Mindful Living Collective is an online community platform where members can connect, share resources, and participate in live events related to mindfulness and meditation.
- Features:
- Live meditation sessions and workshops
- Discussion forums and resource sharing
- Courses on mindfulness, self-compassion, and more
- Why Use It: The interactive and resource-rich environment of the Mindful Living Collective supports ongoing learning and community engagement.

5. MyLife Meditation Community

- Overview: MyLife (formerly Stop, Breathe & Think) offers a

meditation app with personalized recommendations and a community platform for sharing experiences and support.
- Features:
- Personalized meditation recommendations based on your mood
- Guided meditations, breathing exercises, and sleep aids
- Community features for sharing progress and insights
- Why Use It: MyLife's personalized approach and community aspects make it a valuable tool for those seeking tailored meditation guidance and support.

Conclusion

Online courses and communities provide invaluable resources for developing and sustaining a meditation practice. From guided meditations and structured programs to supportive communities and interactive discussions, these platforms offer a wealth of tools to enhance your mindfulness journey. By exploring and engaging with these resources, you can deepen your understanding of meditation, stay motivated, and connect with like-minded individuals, fostering a richer and more fulfilling meditative lifestyle.

Continuing Your Journey

Embarking on a meditation journey is a continuous process of growth, discovery, and deepening awareness. As you progress, you may seek new ways to expand your practice, overcome challenges, and integrate mindfulness more fully into your life. This section provides guidance and resources to help you continue your meditation journey, ensuring that it remains a source of enrichment and transformation.

Exploring Advanced Practices

1. Silent Retreats

- Overview: Silent retreats offer an immersive experience in meditation and mindfulness, typically lasting from a weekend to several weeks. Participants engage in continuous meditation practice, often with guidance from experienced teachers.

- Benefits: Retreats provide an opportunity to deepen your practice, disconnect from daily distractions, and gain profound insights.

- Recommendations:

- Spirit Rock Meditation Center: Located in California, offering retreats led by renowned meditation teachers.

- Insight Meditation Society: Based in Massachusetts, providing silent retreats and intensive meditation courses.

- Plum Village: Founded by Thich Nhat Hanh in France, offering retreats focused on mindfulness and compassionate living.

2. Teacher Training Programs

- Overview: For those interested in teaching meditation or deepening their personal practice, teacher training programs provide comprehensive education in meditation techniques, philosophy, and pedagogy.

- Benefits: Training programs offer a deeper understanding of meditation, enhance personal practice, and prepare individuals to guide others.

- Recommendations:

- Mindfulness-Based Stress Reduction (MBSR) Teacher Training: Offered by the University of Massachusetts Medical School's Center for Mindfulness.

- Search Inside Yourself Leadership Institute (SIYLI): Provides mindfulness and emotional intelligence training.

- Yoga Alliance Certified Meditation Teacher Training: Various yoga schools offer programs that combine yoga and meditation teacher training.

3. Advanced Reading and Study

- Overview: Delving into advanced texts and studies on meditation can provide deeper insights and expand your understanding of the practice.

- Recommendations:

- "The Science of Enlightenment" by Shinzen Young: Explores the intersection of meditation and science.

- "In Love with the World: A Monk's Journey Through the Bardos of Living and Dying" by Yongey Mingyur Rinpoche: A profound exploration of life, death, and meditation.

- "Meditations from the Mat" by Rolf Gates and Katrina Kenison: Combines yoga and meditation insights for a holistic approach.

Engaging with a Community

1. Joining Local Meditation Groups

- Overview: Participating in local meditation groups can provide support, motivation, and a sense of community. These groups often meet regularly for group meditation sessions, discussions, and workshops.

- Benefits: Local groups offer a shared practice environment, opportunities to learn from others, and a supportive network.

- How to Find:

- Search for meditation centers, yoga studios, or spiritual centers in your area.

- Use online platforms like Meetup to find local meditation groups.

2. Online Communities and Forums

- Overview: Online communities provide a space to connect with meditators worldwide, share experiences, and access a wealth of resources.

- Benefits: Online forums offer diverse perspectives, access to international teachers, and support from a global community.

- Recommendations:

- Reddit - r/Meditation: A large, active community discussing various meditation topics.

- Insight Timer Community Groups: Diverse groups within the Insight Timer app for different interests and needs.

- Mindful Living Collective: An online platform for mindfulness practitioners to connect and share resources.

Integrating Meditation into Everyday Life

1. Mindfulness in Daily Activities

- Overview: Continuously integrating mindfulness into daily tasks can transform mundane activities into opportunities for meditation.

- Practices:

- Mindful Eating: Pay full attention to the taste, texture, and aroma of your food.

- Mindful Walking: Focus on the sensation of each step and your breath.

- Mindful Listening: Practice active listening in conversations, giving full attention to the speaker.

2. Creating a Mindful Environment

- Overview: Designing your living and working spaces to promote mindfulness can support your practice.

- Tips:
- Declutter: Keep your environment clean and organized to reduce distractions.
- Nature Elements: Incorporate plants, natural light, and calming colors.
- Mindful Decor: Use artwork, candles, or objects that inspire calm and mindfulness.

Overcoming Challenges and Staying Motivated

1. Addressing Common Obstacles

- Overview: Challenges such as restlessness, doubt, and lack of motivation are common in meditation practice. Developing strategies to overcome these obstacles is crucial for maintaining a consistent practice.
- Strategies:
- Set Realistic Goals: Start with short sessions and gradually increase the duration.
- Practice Self-Compassion: Be kind to yourself and recognize that setbacks are part of the journey.
- Seek Guidance: Consult teachers, mentors, or resources when facing difficulties.

2. Maintaining Motivation

- Overview: Staying motivated can be challenging, especially during periods of stagnation or difficulty. Finding ways to keep your practice engaging and rewarding is essential.
- Tips:
- Regular Reflection: Keep a meditation journal to track your progress and insights.

- Celebrate Milestones: Acknowledge and celebrate your achievements, no matter how small.
- Variety: Explore different meditation techniques and styles to keep your practice fresh and interesting.

Conclusion

Continuing your meditation journey involves exploring advanced practices, engaging with communities, integrating mindfulness into daily life, and overcoming challenges. By utilizing these resources and strategies, you can deepen your practice, maintain motivation, and experience ongoing growth and transformation. Meditation is a lifelong journey, and with dedication and openness, you can continue to cultivate inner peace, clarity, and well-being.

11

Final Conclusion

Reflecting on Your Journey

As you reach the conclusion of this exploration into meditation, it's essential to take a moment to reflect on your journey. Meditation is not merely a practice; it is a path of continuous learning, growth, and self-discovery. Reflecting on your experiences, progress, and the lessons learned along the way can deepen your understanding and appreciation of the transformative power of meditation.

Recognizing Your Progress

1. Acknowledge Milestones

- Reflect on the milestones you've achieved, whether they are small or significant. These can include the first time you meditated, reaching a certain number of consecutive days of practice, or experiencing a moment of profound insight or peace. Recognizing these achievements reinforces your commitment and highlights your progress.

2. Celebrate Growth

- Celebrate the growth you've experienced in your mental, emotional, and spiritual well-being. Notice how your ability to handle stress has improved, how your relationships have deepened, or how you have developed greater self-awareness and compassion. Celebrating these changes can motivate you to continue your practice.

Understanding the Impact

1. Personal Transformation

- Consider how meditation has transformed your life. Reflect on the changes in your perspective, behavior, and overall quality of life. How has meditation helped you navigate challenges, find inner peace, or connect more deeply with yourself and others?

2. Enhanced Well-Being

- Reflect on the physical, mental, and emotional benefits you've experienced. Have you noticed improvements in your health, such as reduced stress or better sleep? Has your mental clarity and focus improved? Do you feel more emotionally balanced and resilient?

Lessons Learned

1. Insights Gained

- Think about the insights and lessons you've gained from your meditation practice. These could be realizations about the nature of your mind, patterns of behavior, or deeper truths about life and existence. How have these insights influenced your daily life and decisions?

2. Challenges Overcome

- Reflect on the challenges you've faced in your meditation journey and how you've overcome them. What strategies or techniques have been most helpful? What have you learned about yourself through these challenges?

Setting Future Intentions

1. Continued Practice

- Set intentions for your continued practice. Consider how you can maintain and deepen your meditation routine. What goals do you have for your practice moving forward? How can you integrate meditation more fully into your daily life?

2. Expanding Horizons

- Explore ways to expand your meditation practice. This might include trying new meditation techniques, attending retreats, or studying more advanced teachings. How can you continue to grow and evolve on your meditation journey?

Embracing the Journey

1. Mindful Living

- Embrace the concept of mindful living, where meditation becomes a way of life rather than a separate activity. Integrate mindfulness into all aspects of your life, from your interactions with others to your daily routines and personal reflections.

2. Lifelong Learning

- Recognize that meditation is a lifelong journey of learning and growth. Approach each session with curiosity and openness, knowing that there is always more to discover and experience.

Conclusion

Reflecting on your meditation journey allows you to appreciate the progress you've made, understand the impact of your practice, and set intentions for the future. Meditation is a path that offers continuous opportunities for growth, insight, and transformation. By acknowledging your achievements, learning from your experiences, and embracing the journey ahead, you can continue to cultivate a deeper sense of mindfulness, inner peace, and well-being. As you move forward, remember that each moment of meditation is a step towards a more mindful, fulfilled, and harmonious life.

The Ongoing Path

Meditation is not a destination but an ongoing path that evolves with you. It is a lifelong journey that offers continuous opportunities for growth, self-discovery, and transformation. As you move forward, it's important to recognize that your practice will change and develop, reflecting your experiences, insights, and life circumstances. This section explores the ongoing nature of the meditation path and how to embrace its dynamic and evolving aspects.

Embracing Change and Growth

1. Adaptability

- Understand that your meditation practice will need to adapt to changes in your life. As you encounter new experiences, challenges, and phases of life, your practice may evolve. Embrace these changes as part of your journey, allowing your practice to grow with you.

2. Continuous Learning

- Maintain a mindset of continuous learning. Meditation offers endless opportunities for exploration and discovery. Stay curious and open to new techniques, philosophies, and insights. This openness will keep your practice fresh and engaging.

3. Self-Compassion

- Practice self-compassion as you navigate the ups and downs of your meditation journey. There will be times when your practice feels easy and fulfilling, and times when it feels challenging or stagnant. Approach each phase with kindness and patience, understanding that each moment is a valuable part of your growth.

Deepening Your Practice

1. Advanced Techniques

- Explore advanced meditation techniques and practices as you become more experienced. Techniques such as Zen meditation, Vipassana, and chakra meditation can offer deeper insights and more profound experiences.

2. Extended Practice

- Consider integrating longer meditation sessions into your routine. Extended practice can help you explore deeper states of consciousness and gain a more comprehensive understanding of your mind and emotions.

3. Retreats and Intensive Practice

- Participate in meditation retreats or intensive practice periods. These immersive experiences provide an opportunity to deepen your practice, disconnect from daily distractions, and connect more fully with your inner self.

Integrating Meditation into Everyday Life

1. Mindful Living

- Strive to make mindfulness a way of life. Integrate mindfulness into all aspects of your daily routine, from mundane tasks to complex interactions. This holistic approach enhances the impact of your practice and fosters a deeper sense of presence and awareness.

2. Relationships and Community

- Share your mindfulness journey with others. Engage with meditation communities, join groups, or participate in discussions. Building connections with like-minded individuals can provide support, inspiration, and a sense of belonging.

3. Service and Compassion

- Use your meditation practice as a foundation for compassionate action. Extend the mindfulness and compassion cultivated in meditation to your interactions with others and your contributions to your community. Acts of service and kindness can deepen your practice and enhance your sense of purpose.

Sustaining Your Practice

1. Regular Review and Reflection

- Periodically review and reflect on your meditation practice. Assess what is working well and what might need adjustment. Reflecting on your journey helps maintain a dynamic and responsive practice.

2. Setting Intentions

- Continuously set intentions for your meditation practice. These intentions can evolve as you grow and change, helping to keep your practice aligned with your current goals and aspirations.

3. Finding Inspiration

- Seek inspiration from various sources to keep your practice vibrant. Read books, listen to talks, attend workshops, and explore different traditions. Inspiration from diverse sources can enrich your practice and provide new perspectives.

Conclusion

The ongoing path of meditation is one of continuous growth, change, and discovery. By embracing adaptability, deepening your practice, integrating mindfulness into everyday life, and sustaining your practice with regular review and inspiration, you can ensure that your meditation journey remains a vital and enriching part of your life. Meditation offers a path to greater mindfulness, inner peace, and well-being that evolves with you, providing endless opportunities for transformation and fulfillment. As you continue on this path, remember to approach each step with curiosity, compassion, and an open heart, knowing that the journey itself is the destination.

Encouragement for the Future

As you continue your meditation journey, it is important to carry forward a sense of encouragement, optimism, and commitment. The practice of meditation is a lifelong endeavor that brings numerous benefits, from improved mental clarity to a deeper sense of inner peace. Here, we offer words of encouragement to inspire and motivate you as you forge ahead on your path.

Embracing the Journey

1. Celebrate Your Efforts

- Acknowledge and celebrate the efforts you've made in your meditation practice. Each moment spent in meditation, every breath taken with mindfulness, and each step towards greater awareness is a significant achievement. Recognize the progress you've made and the commitment you've shown.

2. Stay Open to Growth

- Keep an open heart and mind as you continue your journey. Every experience, whether challenging or uplifting, is an opportunity for growth and learning. Embrace the unknown with curiosity and trust that each step forward is valuable.

Maintaining Motivation

1. Set Meaningful Goals

- Establish meaningful and attainable goals for your meditation practice. Whether it's increasing your daily meditation time, exploring new techniques, or attending a retreat, setting goals can provide direction and motivation.

2. Seek Inspiration

- Continually seek inspiration to fuel your practice. Read books, listen to podcasts, attend workshops, and connect with fellow meditators. Inspiration from various sources can reignite your passion and provide new insights.

3. Practice Patience

- Understand that progress in meditation can be gradual. Be patient with yourself and your practice. Trust that the benefits will unfold over time, and remember that consistency is key to experiencing profound changes.

Building a Supportive Environment

1. Connect with Others

- Engage with meditation communities, both online and in person. Sharing your experiences and learning from others can provide support, encouragement, and a sense of belonging. Surround yourself with individuals who inspire and uplift you.

2. Create a Sacred Space

- Designate a peaceful and inspiring space for your meditation practice. Whether it's a corner of a room or a spot in nature, having a dedicated space can enhance your practice and make it more inviting.

3. Incorporate Rituals

- Establish rituals that support your meditation practice. Simple actions like lighting a candle, playing calming music, or reciting an affirmation can signal to your mind and body that it's time to meditate, creating a sense of sacredness around your practice.

Fostering Resilience

1. Embrace Challenges

- View challenges as integral parts of your meditation journey. Each obstacle is an opportunity to strengthen your resilience and deepen your understanding. Embrace these moments with a mindset of growth and learning.

2. Cultivate Self-Compassion

- Practice self-compassion in your meditation and daily life. Be gentle with yourself, especially during difficult times. Recognize that everyone faces challenges and that self-kindness is a powerful tool for overcoming them.

3. Stay Committed

- Commit to your practice with determination and dedication. Remind yourself of the reasons you began this journey and the benefits you've experienced. Let your commitment to personal growth and well-being guide you through any difficulties.

Looking Ahead

1. Lifelong Journey

- Remember that meditation is a lifelong journey. There is no final destination, only continuous exploration and discovery. Embrace the path with a sense of adventure and openness, knowing that each step brings new insights and deeper understanding.

2. Impact on Your Life

- Reflect on how meditation has already impacted your life and imagine the possibilities for the future. Envision how continued practice can further enhance your well-being, relationships, and overall sense of purpose.

3. Share Your Practice

- Consider sharing the benefits of meditation with others. Teaching or introducing friends and family to meditation can reinforce your practice and create a ripple effect of mindfulness and peace in your community.

Conclusion

As you move forward, carry these words of encouragement with you. The journey of meditation is rich with opportunities for growth, learning, and transformation. Embrace each moment with an open heart, stay committed to your practice, and trust in the profound benefits that meditation can bring to your life. Your dedication to this path is a testament to your desire for inner peace and well-being, and each step you take is a step towards a more mindful and fulfilling life. Keep going with confidence and curiosity, knowing that the journey itself is the reward.